When Simple Becomes Extraordinary

A 60-year-old diabetic man's journey
from 28 years of sedentary living
to ultramarathon finisher

Robert F. Schuler

Foreword by Matt Fitzgerald, Author of *80/20 Running*
Edited by Ted Griffin

1st Edition
Published by L&R Media LLC

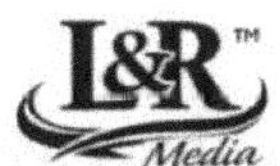

Published by L&R Media LLC
L&R Media LLC, 200 N. High St., P.O. Box 421,
Canal Winchester, OH 43110

Library of Congress Control Number: 2026905136
ISBN 979-8-9949925-0-0 (paperback)

Printed in the United States of America

Cover design and interior by Robert F. Schuler

With appreciation for their love and support, I dedicate this book to my wife and adult children, without whose encouragement this book would have no content.

Table of Contents

Preface

It was in March, 2024, shortly after my sixty-second birthday, while on a scheduled morning run, that I agreed to listen to the voice in my head telling me to write down the events of my physical training over the previous two years. I managed to push away this "whispering" for several months, choosing to focus on doing, rather than talking about what was already done. At this point, I completed over three hundred morning runs and seventeen chip-timed races. The mile count was over fifteen hundred.

As I continued on my run in the cool March air, a persuasive thought repeated in my mind, *If I was able to maintain this exercise program starting at sixty years old, how many others could follow the same (or similar) steps and receive the benefits that I found?*

David Mathis, in his book, "A Little Theology of Exercise," states, "Alongside breathing, eating, thinking, feeling, and speaking, one of the great fundamentals of human life is movement" (Mathis, 2025, p. 8). Mathis adds that "many people just want to take pills. Few want to take exercise. The prescription may be simple, but it's not easy" (Mathis, 2025, p. 59).

According to the Centers for Disease Control and Prevention (CDC), over 38 million people in the United States have type-2 diabetes, which is over 10% of the population. Type-2 diabetes most often develops in people forty-five or older who are less physically active. Additionally; Type-2 diabetes can be prevented with proven lifestyle changes that include losing weight, choosing a healthy diet, and getting regular physical activity (CDC, 2024).

These days; people are living longer (U.S. Census Bureau, 2018). When combined with the large number of people born in the baby-boomer generation, the U.S. is facing the largest ever distribution of people living over the age of sixty. As people age, so grows the instance of common health challenges, such as; cardiovascular disease, cancer, diabetes, hypertension, age-related muscle loss (also called senescence), and osteoporosis (bone density loss) (Woolf & Schoomaker, 2019). Other common concerns tied to aging include, malnutrition, dehydration, cognitive decline, and reduced physical activity, or sedentary living, which leads to muscle atrophy, weakness, and chronic pain (He & Sharpless, 2017).

This information raised questions in my mind. *Are the above ailments simply part of growing old? Was I destined to accept declines in my health as I aged? Are older adults powerless to do anything to counteract this decline?*

In this book; I will share how twenty-eight years of sedentary living affected my life. I will share how I discovered a new lifestyle, based on a simple progressive plan of daily movement that included replacing limiting beliefs with consistent action and accomplishment.

Twenty-eight years is a long time. It totals over 10,000 days. As the subtitle of this book states, that is the length of time that I lived a mostly sedentary lifestyle. When I think back, each individual year seemed to pass very quickly. Most people would agree that it is astonishing how fast time flies. I was always busy with work, teaming up with my wife to parent our four children, or chasing after other responsibilities.

Over the years I attempted many exercise programs, often tied to a New Year's resolution. Starting was easy for me. Continuing was hard. Choosing to skip a day was the norm— and then skip again. I often thought, *I'll exercise tomorrow.* My procrastination piled up thousands of tomorrows that turned into yesterdays while my health gradually declined, eventually leading to type-2 diabetes, high cholesterol, and near obesity.

This book details my journey of discovery to improved health, a new understanding of key systems of the body, and simple steps to sustainable and consistent exercise.

Foreword

Here's a tip: If you want to learn how to sing as an adult, don't take lessons from an instructor with perfect pitch. Having never known what it's like to sing off-key, these natural-born songbirds won't relate to your struggles, nor will you relate to their fluid ease with vocal expression.

Likewise, I'm not the best guy to inspire out-of-shape adults to get moving and enjoy the many benefits of an active lifestyle. The son of a Navy SEAL turned marathoner, I started running at age eleven and haven't stopped. For me, running is as natural as hitting the right notes is for the singer with perfect pitch. As much as I love welcoming new members into the community of runners, I have a hard time relating to the struggles most people face when they start out later in life.

Bobby Schuler does not. As you will learn in reading this inspiring and important book, Bobby did not become a regular exerciser of any kind, much less an ultramarathon runner, until he was past his sixtieth birthday. Every challenge you can imagine facing as a late-life beginner Bobby has faced, from the life-changing medical diagnosis that scared him into attempting those humbling first workouts to the aches and pains he experienced trying to get out of bed the next morning.

No matter who you are, I'm confident you will see something of yourself in Bobby—at least in the beginning. But will you still find him relatable when he runs a half marathon, and then a marathon, and then an ultramarathon—something that less that one in ten thousand people ever does? I think you will.

That's the magic of When Simple Becomes Extraordinary: Through the power of story it makes the impossible seem possible. Bobby Schuler is the same ordinary guy from the beginning of the story all the way to the end; yet he goes from living an ordinary life to doing extraordinary things. And by the time you put this book down you'll be thinking, "Heck, if he can do it, I can too!" And you're right; you can!

But that doesn't mean you will. It all depends on whether you fall in love with running or some other form of exercise, as Bobby did. You see, people start exercising for a lot of reasons—health scares, weight-loss goals, stress reduction, and so forth—but the number-one reason people keep exercising once they've started is enjoyment. And the best way to learn to enjoy exercise, as Bobby learned, is to become an athlete.

"It was much more enjoyable to be training to compete against others and myself," he observes while preparing for his first race, "rather than just exercising because I was following the advice of my doctor." Truer words were never spoken.

All of the health benefits Bobby has earned by becoming more active are secondary to his discovery of a passion for physical exertion. Your chances of earning the same benefits will be far greater if you discover the same passion, and there's something about crossing a finish line with a number on your belly that instills a hunger for more. It might not make sense to you now, but it will when you get there.

Until then, let me get out of your way and let Bobby work his magic, simple but extraordinary.

Matt Fitzgerald, running coach and author of more than thirty books on health and fitness

Introduction

It was Sunday, February 2, 2014. I settled into my place as the first quarter of Super Bowl XLVIII (48) was underway. The teams were the Seattle Seahawks and the Denver Broncos, playing in MetLife Stadium located in East Rutherford, New Jersey. This stadium has no roof or dome. It was the first Super Bowl to be played in an open-air, cold-climate city. I possessed little knowledge of the Seahawks or the Broncos apart from both teams posting a 13-3 record during the regular season. I didn't favor one team over the other. I just wanted to watch championship-level football. Then came the distraction.

RING!! What? Someone was calling my mobile phone from an unknown number during the game. I promptly declined the call, sending the "interrupter" directly to voicemail. BING. My phone dinged, indicating a new voicemail. Okay, the person seemed to have a purpose for calling me or was a persistent telemarketer. I called into my voicemail and listened. It was my doctor. I listened to the message, "Hello Mr. Schuler. It's not an emergency, but *[slight pause]* I need you to call me back as soon as you listen to this message." While his words stated no emergency, they carried an obvious urgency. I called him back.

"Mr. Schuler, thanks for returning my call. I received your test results and your blood glucose and cholesterol numbers are quite elevated. Your glucose is 286 and your A1C is 8.2. You have type-2 diabetes."

The doctor went on to explain that type-2 diabetes occurs when the blood glucose (B/G) reading is above the normal range of 70 to 120 and A1C is above the normal range of 4.0 and 5.6 (with A1C being the average percentage of glucose in the blood over the previous 90 days) (Tinfang, 2014).

The doctor explained that it was best that I start on medications right away, along with urging me to lose weight and begin regular, weekly physical exercise. He suggested I start by walking more. Simple ways to do this included; skip the elevator and take the stairs, park your car farther from the office or store, and walk (or ride a bike) to the train station (Tinfang, 2014).

After hanging up the phone, I took a deep breath as the gravity of the call hit me. This was a serious wake-up call! I informed my wife and daughter and suddenly lost all interest in the Super Bowl.

Over the coming days I began researching the inner-workings of the hormone **insulin** on blood sugar. Insulin is released by the pancreas and acts as a delivery agent of the glucose in the blood, which, when received in the cells, is converted into energy for thc various systems of the body. With type-2 diabetics, cells of the body resist the delivery of glucose by insulin, which is referred to as **insulin resistance** (Merriam-Webster's Medical Dictionary, 2016). As glucose remains in the blood stream, it eventually crystallizes, which causes damage to various parts of the body, including blood vessels, eyes, nerves, feet and in severe cases, can cause limb amputations, kidney failure, strokes, and heart disease (National Kidney Foundation, 2014). My weight at the time was 184, which was down from my all-time high of 196, and my pant size was a tight-fitting 36-30. Being five feet seven inches tall, these numbers straddled below and above the obesity line, according to the **body mass index** (BMI). BMI is a widely accepted, general

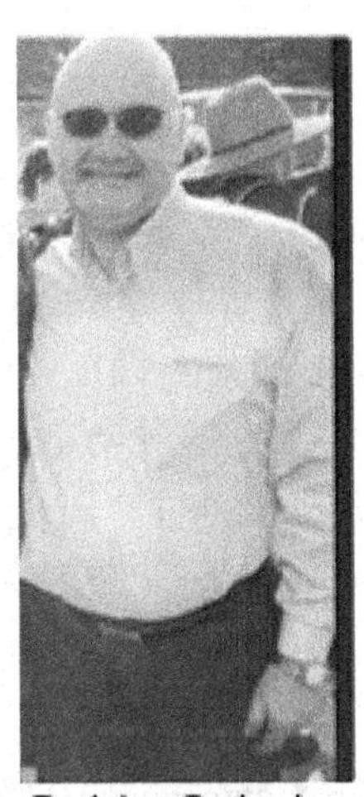

Bobby Schuler in 2014

measurement of health and is calculated by dividing body weight (in kilograms) by the square of body height (in meters) (Merriam-Webster's Medical Dictionary, 2016). When I was in high school (thirty-five years earlier), I weighed 144 with a waist-inseam pant size of 30-30. Boy-o-boy, were those days long gone! The top of normal on the BMI range for my height is 159; so it was prudent that I lose a minimum of 25 pounds.

The following week I joined a local gym and spent most of my time on an elliptical machine, with the goal to gradually raise my heart rate (HR) while keeping impact on my joints to a minimum. Since early childhood I have always loved bike riding; so I bought a used cruiser bike. This bike is designed with the pedals slightly forward in relationship to the seat, creating a posture-friendly, sit-tall, riding experience. Cruisers are designed to provide a pleasant, low-exertion ride.

During this time my exercise schedule could be best described as haphazard. Some weeks included four to six exercise sessions, while others didn't have any. With this mild level of exercise and taking the daily medications, my A1C dropped to 7.4. I was going in the right direction, but I was still above the type-2 diabetes A1C measurement line of 6.5. I found myself questioning the engrained, regular habit of buying a candy bar. When someone asked me if I had a sweet tooth I would say, "No, all my teeth are sweet, not just one." Despite lowering my sugar intake and my less frequent inconsistent exercise, my early morning B/G reading at this time was mostly in the 140s, but occasionally as high as 160. Something inside me knew that I needed a more consistent approach to physical exercise, one that would effectively address my insulin resistance.

From 2014 through 2016 my career took some abrupt turns, causing us to move a few times, with the last move bringing us to Columbus, Ohio. In 2017 I began to settle into my new surroundings and became very interested in the sport of golf. There was a nice 18-hole course located less than ten minutes from my home, which became a regular place for me to play. I mostly hit balls at the driving range, with an occasional stint at playing nine holes on the course. While I found golf to be lots of fun, the only aspect of the sport to raise my HR was when I made an errant tee shot that made contact with a home located along the fairway. That's not the kind of high HR that brings health.

By 2021 I was mostly riding my cruiser bike in and around my neighborhood for structured exercise. While the cruiser was great for helping me move in general, it was not the best for raising my HR in a sustained fashion. I decided to look online for a used road bike. Unlike a cruiser, a road bike is designed for speed and an aerodynamic ride.

I found a used road bike that was about 10 years old, but in good condition. Wow, was it different when compared to the cruiser. The road bike had a light-weight frame with a high seat and a low handlebar. The controls were built into the handle grips, giving the rider instant access to all 24 gears and both front and rear brakes. To me this bike was like a high-performance race car.

It took me a little time to figure out how to up- and down-shift, but once I did, riding this bike was a delight. Since it was a used bike, I decided to take it to my local shop for a tune up. After tuning, all the gears shifted as smooth as silk. The level of resistance between gears was subtle, which allowed me to control both the speed and the level of effort to a high degree. Acceleration was insanely quick. Compared to the cruiser, this was like a mechanical retelling of the story of the tortoise and the hare.

After doing some online research I learned that many road bikes are fitted with special pedals called clip-ins. Clip-ins are pedals that work with specifically designed shoes that have a medal clip on the sole that attaches into a similar clip on each pedal. This allows the rider to generate continual forward energy even with each up-stroke of the legs because the shoes are locked into the pedals. When a rider needs to remove his feet, he rotates his foot about 15° to release the shoe from the clip (this is also called, clipping-out). The task of clipping-out can be tricky, especially when the pedals are new, because the springs that hold the clips in place are new and tight.

Before my first ride I practiced clipping-in and clipping-out. It seemed easy enough. So I started a nice, slow ride on a side street with very little car traffic. I decided to pull over to a near-by curb, slowing to a gentle stop. I attempted to clip-out, but my right shoe would not release. Subsequently a helpless feeling waved over me as my feet remained in the pedals and the "stopped" bike slowly tipped over into the grass. Over the next couple of weeks and with a lot more practice, I developed better skill clipping out.

The following Saturday morning, I was riding on a nearby bike path and I did not see a speed bump at an intersection. Speed bumps are usually marked with yellow or white street paint so drivers and riders can clearly see them. This speed bump did not have any paint. I was riding at a moderate speed (maybe 12 mph), when my front tire hit the bump. The bike immediately went airborne. I recall the feeling of slow motion for a very long couple of seconds, and then I and the bike hit the pavement HARD! The crash resulted in no damage to the bike, other than the front handle bar being a little bent (which was easily straightened). I, on the other hand, was another story.

I saw blood coming from a knee, and my shoulder was radiating moderate pain, being the first part of my body to make contact with the ground. I noticed a few other bumps and bruises. I took a deep breath and thanked the Good Lord that I was not badly injured. I thought, *Okay, I need to do a much better job of watching the road.* I decided to look for paths without any speed bumps and to buy a set of rubberized knee protectors.

I shared the crash story with my son, and he suggested that I consider using an indoor bike trainer. A bike trainer is a device that the rear wheel fits into, allowing riding inside while still utilizing all the features of the bike (e.g., the clip-in pedals and gear shifting). Some bike trainers have very fancy features, including computerized programs of biking destinations all over the world that are projected onto a tablet or other screen, and are coded into the trainer so that when the screen shows a hill, the trainer causes the rider to feel a simulated incline. I opted for a simple, non-computerized trainer that fit in my budget of $100 or less. I later discovered (and purchased) a $20 bluetooth bike sensor that attaches to the axle of my rear wheel and would measure my speed and total distance through an app on my smartphone. Once the trainer was set up I felt free to go as fast as I wanted without the fear of crashing. I didn't need to clip-out or watch for cars, pedestrians, or speed bumps.

Early on another Saturday morning I decided to find out what the effect would be on my B/G number if I rode 17 miles in one hour on the trainer. It was physically grueling. I completed the distance only by pushing my speed past 20 mph for the last several minutes. After the ride I checked my B/G number, and it was only 20 points lower than my reading first thing that morning. I was shocked!! I wondered why my number didn't go lower after such a maximum effort. I paused and began to consider other forms of exercise that would hopefully make a more demonstrative impact on lowering my B/G number.

The next Saturday I decided to try running. Following a cup of coffee, I grabbed a pair of shorts and ventured out to the street by my home. I started with a very gentle jog, and after about half a block I was out of breath and could feel my heart nearly beating out of my chest. I slowed to a walk to allow my heart to recover. I continued this run-walk until I completed a lap around my neighborhood, which turned out to be just short of a mile. Even though it was less than one mile, I felt very spent from this short time jogging. It was super-obvious that my cardiorespiratory fitness level was very low.

After returning to my home I took a B/G reading and could hardly believe my eyes. My number was over 40 points lower than my initial morning reading about an hour earlier. This little "run" took less than 15 minutes and accomplished more to lower my B/G number than the vigorous 17-mile bike ride! *Okay, I'm giving running an equal voice from now on*, I thought.

A couple weeks later, in early August 2021, over my morning coffee I thought about registering for a race. This would add a competitive element to my exercise. In the summer of 2009 my son participated in the Chicago Triathlon. A triathlon is a three-phase race that involves three exercise disciplines: swimming, bike riding, and running. My son registered for the Olympic distance; which is a 1.5 kilometer (K; 0.93 of a mile) swim in Lake Michigan, followed by a 40K bike ride (24.8 miles) on the center lanes of Lake Shore Drive, and finishing with a 10K (6.2 mile) run on the Chicago Lakefront Trail.

Throughout my life I was never much of a swimmer. While my eighth-grade buddies from school were doing swan dives off the three-meter springboard at our local pool, I managed, after much coaxing by those same buddies, to jump off the one-meter board into 12 feet of alarmingly deep water. I identified with the fear that Chief Brody suffered in the 1975 movie *Jaws*. During the dinner scene Mrs. Brody explained to Mr. Hooper that Chief Brody had hated the water since childhood. She asked if there was a clinical name for it, and Chief Brody provided the one-word response, "Drowning" (Spielberg et al., 2012, 0:42:20–0:42:33).

So with swimming off the table for the time being, I grabbed my phone and typed the words, "triathlon without swimming" into an Internet search. The search returned something called a duathlon. I thought, *What in the world is a duathlon?*

A duathlon is a three-phase race that deploys two exercise disciplines with one of the disciplines repeating. Instead of the three different disciplines of a triathlon, a duathlon repeats one discipline (run-bike-run). *This was it!*, I thought. I performed another search for duathlon races in my area and discovered the *Ohio Fall Challenge,* scheduled on September 26, 2021. This was an event hosting multiple distances for both the triathlon and the duathlon. Hundreds of people were registered to participate. I decided to sign up for the mini-duathlon (also called the Mini-Du). This race is comprised of a two-mile run, a seven-mile ride, and a two-mile run. I had just under eight weeks to train for it.

Train? Yes, train! That word sounded different in my mind. There's something official, even athletic, about the word. My exercise now had a purpose that could be objectively measured through competition with others. At the time I didn't consider myself an athlete. My mind was now opening to the possibility of developing athletic ability. As I pondered the race I could feel a subtle, quiet excitement beginning to build.

Part I: When Humility Becomes Hope

1. Preparing for the Duathlon

As I ventured into the world of running, I knew very little about running form or how to train. I began searching for reading material and set aside any preconceived notions, opening my mind to find 21st-century publications and writings on the sport.

The last time I bought a pair of running shoes was during my junior year of high school, 42 years earlier. I asked some peers at work where they thought I should start. One peer strongly suggested I go to a particular running shoe store. He told me they would scan my feet to understand the pressure points where my feet make contact with the ground and ask me to run a bit on their treadmill. This process is called analysis of the running **gait**, which is used to observe the pattern of movement when someone walks or runs (Merriam-Webster, 2020).

A comprehensive gait analysis not only includes observing where each foot strikes the ground in relation to the body, but looks for the alignment of the hips, knees, and ankles, in order to see if any muscle imbalances exist. Pronation or supination at the ankle joint can be present during walking or running. If a muscle imbalance is observed, then the evaluator uses this information to recommend the type of running shoe that best addresses that muscle imbalance (Sutton, 2022, p. 197).

I followed my peer's advice and went to that running shoe store, underwent their standard analysis, and then tried on several different shoes that the sales person recommended. I settled on a pair of shoes that felt like cushioned pillows under my feet. The sales person called them daily trainers. All I knew was, these running shoes were the most comfortable shoes I had worn in many years.

My Assessment of Race Readiness

As I began running on the street in these new shoes, I started to feel an ache in my shins on both legs. I remembered experiencing this ache at different times in my life when running and I knew what it was. Shin splints! I searched online and found a post that advised taking a walk break whenever feeling my shins aching, and when the ache subsides, resume running. In the first few days of trying this, I was alternating between running and walking about every twenty steps. It seemed ridiculous, but I soldiered on, and after about two weeks, the ache from the shin splints completely stopped and did not return.

During these early days I could still only run about half a block, and my HR would climb to 160. This number was still very high for such a gentle, short run. I decided to search for beginner books on running and found a book written by Matt Fitzgerald titled, *80/20 Running*. The first five chapters of Fitzgerald's book blew up everything I thought I knew about building cardiorespiratory fitness. The book thoroughly demonstrates how slow running at low intensity 80% of the time is a proven way to build base cardiorespiratory fitness (Fitzgerald, 2014, p. 1-100).

Learning that I did not need to push myself hard on my runs was a great relief. Even when I ran slow, my HR was very high; so I realized I needed to allow walk breaks to bring it down. At the time I owned a smart watch, which tracked my HR from a wrist sensor. Using a watch to monitor my HR reminded me of an experience about ten years earlier when I signed up for a fitness boot camp offered by my employer during the lunch hour.

The Fitness Boot Camp

This company provided employees with an on-site fitness facility equipped with cardio machines, free weights, and personal trainers. I was told by a peer worker that the bootcamp is very tough. Armed with this info, I decided to use an HR monitor watch and chest strap that I purchased years earlier (but sat in a drawer most of the time).

As a warmup the instructor directed us to run around some cones he setup that seemed to be about a 200-meter (an eighth of a mile) loop. After the first loop I was out of breath and trailing at the rear of the other dozen participants. It wasn't long before my watch started beeping, signaling that I had exceeded 100% of my Max HR. According to the watch manual, Max HR is a calculation that the watch makes by subtracting the wearer's age from 220. This meant that my Max HR at the time was 168 (220 - 52 = 168). Max HR is commonly used in training to determine five HR exercise zones by subtracting a certain percentage from the Max HR.

After the warmup run concluded, the instructor explained the next set of workout activities. During his talk my watch never stopped beeping (indicating that my HR was still elevated from the warm up run). Finally he asked, "What is that beeping?" I told him it was my watch indicating that my heart was about to explode. The instructor told me to sit out on additional exercises until the watch stopped beeping. All kidding aside, the bootcamp was very tough indeed, confirming my peer's earlier feedback.

Looking back, it would have been wise for me to complete a health risk assessment prior to joining the bootcamp. A **health risk assessment** (HRA) is "a screening tool used to evaluate the benefits and the risks associated with starting any type of exercise that is strenuous in nature" (Sutton, 2022, p, 342-344). An HRA is a review by a fitness professional of the current physical activity of an individual that includes checking his ability to perform basic range-of-motion (ROM) movements for limbs and joints and perhaps most importantly a review of his cardiorespiratory fitness. Had I taken an HRA, it is very likely that I would have been advised to opt for a lower-intensity training program rather than the rigors of the bootcamp.

It is always a good idea to check with your primary-care physician before starting any fitness program, especially if you know the program will be pushing your limits. I attempted a couple more sessions of the bootcamp, but then decided it was best to withdraw.

Training Before the Duathlon

With the shin splints solved and my smart watch tracking my heart, I embarked on early-morning training runs before work. I completed over 20 training runs from August 20, 2021 through September 24, 2021. These runs varied up to four miles. During each training run I kept an eye on my heart rate.

From my short time in the fitness bootcamp, I recalled the instructor asking us to rate from 1 to 10 how hard we felt we were working on an exercise, with 1 being the easiest and 10 being the hardest. He called this, **relative perceived exertion** (RPE). During these early runs I rarely felt any run was below a 7 on the RPE scale. As an added measurement, if my HR number on my watch went above 160, I walked until it was below 130. Toward the end of September, I was as ready as I could be before race day.

What I liked the most about training was my new purpose of preparing for a race. It was much more enjoyable to be training to compete against others and myself rather than just exercising because I was following the advice of my doctor. Preparing for a public race validated all the work I was putting into my training and I was eager to see how I would perform during the race.

2. Duathlon Race Day

I woke early on Saturday, September 26, 2021. The race location was in Deer Creek State Park, on the edge of Deer Creek Lake, with a start time of 8:00 A.M. The drive was about fifty minutes, mostly on narrow two-lane roads. I decided to depart early enough in order to arrive no later than 7:00 A.M. to receive my race packet and find a spot to setup my bike and running gear.

After checking my glucose numbers, drinking some coffee, and making a quick stop in the bathroom, I was ready to depart. I had loaded the car the night before and made a quick equipment check to confirm that everything was loaded. I mounted my phone in the dash-holder with the destination entered into the GPS and eased my CR-V into the darkness just before 6:00 A.M.

It wasn't long before I was on one of those narrow roads that ran between two large corn fields. The only light was coming from my high-beams, which were perpetually engaged, except when I saw an oncoming car. Were it not for the GPS, heaven only knows where I would have ended up! The estimated arrival time was spot-on. A great feeling of relief waved over me when I saw a sign with the event logo and a big arrow pointing to the parking area. I pulled into a spot after driving past dozens of cars, trucks, and SUV's, most of which had all types of bikes mounted in every way imaginable. After parking, I walked over to the registration area and received my race packet and thought to myself, *There is no turning back now. I'm doing this!*

Butterflies

As I looked through my race packet, I found my chipped bib (the waterproof paper that shows the registered race number), an event t-shirt, and miscellaneous marketing items from race sponsors. I unloaded the bike, grabbed my duffle bag with my running shoes, and headed over to the bike transition area. I found a nice spot right by a fence and noticed that some folks were tying bandannas or handkerchiefs to the fence to make their bike easier to find after the first run phase; so I tied a plastic bag to the fence adjacent to my bike location.

Once all my gear and bike were situated, I put on my rubber knee supports and running shoes. It was 7:45 A.M. and the phase-1 run would be starting soon. As I walked over to the starting area, I felt butterflies like I never had before. I thought to myself, *Schuler, you trained a bunch for this! You can do it. Just take a deep breath and calm down!* At the starting area I saw every age group from teens to what I assumed were folks in their forties, but did not see anyone near my age.

Phase 1 (two mile run)

A man who was clearly part of the race administration asked everyone to remove their hats for the playing of the National Anthem – which he played on a portable boombox. After the anthem he gave us some simple instructions on the turns during the run, along with an intersection we were required to cross during the bike portion. He then told us the race would start at the sound of his hand-held horn. Within five seconds, we heard the horn, and we were running.

During the first mile I noticed that all the butterflies disappeared as soon as I started running. My running pace during the race was definitely faster than the pace I ran during my training. I would find out later that this is a classic rookie mistake, allowing the race atmosphere and/or other runners to influence my pace. On the other hand I didn't really have a pace in mind–another rookie mistake. In any event I maintained this fast pace until I glanced at my watch and noticed that my HR was over 170. I never saw a number that high at any point in my training. I slowed to a brisk walk to allow my HR to come down. It took several minutes, but then I thought, *It's only two miles;* so I resumed running, but at a slower pace. The course took a turn into a dead-end street that we looped in and then out again. This loop was used only going out and then was skipped on the way back to the finish line.

With my HR lower now, I resumed the earlier faster pace and completed the run. The finish line was located adjacent to the bike transition area. I was not certain if I should go directly to my bike or cross the finish line first and then go to my bike. I decided to cross the finish line first and then back-tracked to the bike transition area. I later found out that proceeding directly to my bike after the first phase was correct. I eventually located my bike and changed out of my running shoes and into the bike clip-in shoes. Riders were not permitted to mount their bike in the transition area, to reduce the chance of runner-rider collisions; so I walked my bike to the starting area for the ride.

Phase 2 (seven mile ride)

In the starting area I mounted my bike with my left foot clipped in and my right foot on the ground. It was probably a survival instinct that I decided to clip-in only the left foot, so that I had my right foot free. My bike didn't come with triathlon bars (aka tri-bars). Tri-bars are used to allow the rider to stay in a very low, tucked position for the purpose of reducing wind resistance. A couple of weeks earlier I had purchased a pair of do-it-yourself tri-bars that screwed onto the center of my handle bar. This created a bit of a quandary for me, as my gear-shifters and brakes were mounted to the standard bar. I investigated moving the brake and gear-shift cables from the standard bar to the tri-bars, but it was not feasible. When I used the tri-bars, if I wanted to change gears or break I needed to transition my hand down from the tri-bars to the standard bar. If I wasn't careful, the movement of my hand from the tri-bar to the standard bar could upset the center of balance of the front wheel and possibly cause me to crash. Because of this risk, I elected not to use the tri-bars during the race.

As the ride progressed, I saw a teenager way ahead of everyone else in the race. What I didn't know was, multiple riders from other races were riding the course together with us mini-duer's. Some of those riders looked like they were riding bikes that were more expensive than my car. As I was approaching the 3.5 mile turn-about (i.e., the halfway point), one of those riders came alongside me to pass me. His bike was so quiet that I didn't even hear him approaching. As he passed, he was so close that his right shoulder nearly brushed my left shoulder. Being startled, I said, "Whoa!" He smiled, not saying a word as he continued passing me. It became apparent to me that he was racing one of the longer courses because he did not take the Mini-Du turn-around.

A few minutes later I noticed the earlier teenager was now riding toward me and back to the transition area, maintaining his significant lead. I saw a couple of other teen riders a couple hundred meters ahead of me; so I sped up and passed them. I decided to stop changing gears and settled into a steady pedal cadence that yielded about 16 mph. Before I knew it, I was pulling into the transition area for the final run phase.

Phase 3 (two mile run)

I found my spot in the transition area, changed into my running shoes as fast as I could, and headed back out. I quickly realized that my energy level was noticeably lower compared to the earlier run, with my heart exceeding 170 beats a lot faster than the first time. I walked for about a block and then resumed a slower run pace, which would be more accurately called a jog. I remembered the route from earlier and pushed a faster pace, but my lungs and heart were not in agreement. Over the next half mile I switched between running and walking about every thirty steps. I was on my way back to the finish line and for some unknown reason I decided to cross the street and run into the dead-end loop. About 150 feet into the loop I realized the error and turned back. This detour added two or three minutes to my time. As I approached the finish line a new feeling of accomplishment flooded over me. I did it! It was not a long race, but it was my first race, and it was officially in the books.

Race Results

After crossing the finish line, I walked over to the area where the race administration team mounted screens with the real-time results. I found my name listed on the screen. I placed eleventh out of a total of thirty-three participants. My transition times, the time taken while moving from run-to-ride and ride-to-run, were among the slowest of all the participants.

The teenager who I saw in the lead won the race with an overall time of 49 minutes 16 seconds (49:16 in race time format). His average minutes per mile (MPM) for the two run portions were 5:31 and 5:58 respectively. He averaged 17.3 mph on the bike. My pace for the run portions were 9:34 MPM and 11:01 MPM, with my ride averaging 15.6 mph (Triregistration.com, 2021). I was surprised by how much faster my run times were when compared to my training runs. The competitive race environment definitely played a part in my running faster.

After seeing my results, I loaded my bike and gear in my car, then walked over to watch some bikers in the transition area finishing longer races. I saw one woman release the clips on her shoes and pulled her feet out of her clip-in shoes while leaving the shoes in the pedals. She then proceeded to run with stocking feet through the transition area. I mentioned it to a gentleman standing near me.

"She left her shoes in the pedals."

He replied, "I did too! It saved me a couple of seconds. Every second counts!"

As I nodded in response I thought, *These folks care about two seconds? They are very competitive!!*

All in all I felt good about my first race. I learned things that can only be learned through participation in an event; like how close some bikers ride to other bikers, the importance of moving quickly through the transition area, and staying on the course. Finishing in eleventh place overall was better than I expected. The two things I enjoyed most were, (1) learning that I could finish a race, and (2) discovering that competing in a race was a whole lot of fun!

Part II: When Difficult Becomes Determination

3. Setting a Daunting Goal

fter finishing the mini-duathlon race I was ready to start looking for another goal and another race. As I pondered what goal I should reach for, I began thinking about cycling in races:

Do I like races that include cycling? To be a competitive cyclist, I would need to ride fast. Cycling fast adds a risk of crashing and injury. What if I just focused on running?

The answer to these questions, I was soon to discover, would have to wait.

Work and Health Challenges

In the closing months of 2021 I was working as a remote technology procurement consultant. The projects I worked on involved negotiating purchase contracts for technology products and services.

Shortly after completing the duathlon my workload rose substantially, with several projects all needing to be completed by the end of the calendar year.

My wife worked as a teacher and librarian in a nearby grade school. In early September the morning air temperatures where we live are cooler, but rise above 70° Fahrenheit in the afternoon. These cold and hot swings invariably cause children in the school to become ill. Once that happens the colds, coughs, and other illnesses can spread through the school quickly, with all the teachers and staff right in the middle of it. It is a common thing for my wife and me to catch whatever illness is passing through the school. Between October 2021 and March 2022, with my heavy workload and my wife and me battling a number of illnesses that passed through the school, I was not able to carve out much time for running.

Final Decision on Bike Races

With the arrival of spring, 2022 my health finally improved enough for me to begin thinking about my next running goal and race. I settled in my mind, for the time being, that I would not participate in races that included a cycling element.

I was introduced to a new term, cross-training. Cross-training is an exercise session that is different from one's primary sport or activity and is intended to assist the body with recovery (Higdon, 2016, p.150). For me, running is my primary sport; so I decided that when I rode my bike it would be for the purpose of cross-training.

The Columbus Half Marathon

I began my search for a challenging, run-only event scheduled in late summer or autumn. One such event was the Columbus Half Marathon. This race was scheduled on October 16, 2022 and was a combined event with the Columbus Marathon. The longest run that I completed up to this point was seven miles, when I was a teenager. Completing my first half marathon at the age of sixty definitely qualified as challenge enough.

I noticed different running groups on social media posting training plans. I did not have a training plan for the mini-du. I didn't have any plan at all. I just went out to run and ride. I wondered if I needed a training plan for the half marathon. Then the words of a VP I used to work for came to mind: *If you fail to plan, you are planning to fail.*

Finding a Beginner Training Plan

After a short search online I found a beginner book that would help me, *Hal Higdon's Half Marathon Training* (Higdon, 2016). Before buying his book I performed an Internet search on Mr. Higdon and discovered that he is a former elite runner, who completed 111 marathons in his lifetime, including a 2:29 marathon at the age of 49, which translates to 5:43 MPM (Higdon, 2025). This was encouraging to me because I was keen on finding a plan that I could execute as a 60-year-old with virtually no running experience.

After receiving the book I immediately looked through the Table of Contents and turned to the page with beginner training plans. Hal called them "novice training programs," and he included two in the book. They both included something called a long run. The long run is completed at an easy running pace and focuses on building endurance. Each week the long run distance is increased over the previous week, with the last long run of the plan approaching the race distance. As defined by Hal, the long run is "the most important workout of the week" because of the progression of longer distances. It is common that the longest long run is shorter than the full distance of the race, so as not to burnout the runner. The thought of running all those miles in training made me wonder if I did (or did not) have what it takes to complete a race of this magnitude (Higdon, 2016, p, 108).

Finalizing the Training Plan

The training plan I settled on was 12 weeks in length. With the current date in early June, the Columbus Half Marathon was 19 weeks away. So I took the plan and counted backward twelve weeks from the race date. I decided that the initial seven weeks would repeat the first week of the plan, with the long run for that week being four miles. With my run fitness level still low I could use these weeks to get accustomed to following a plan day after day and week after week without too much concern about long distances.

I created a spreadsheet for the plan, with the days of the week in columns across the top, starting with Monday through Sunday. Each week was listed on two rows to include the planned run distance and actual miles completed. The date column represents the Monday date for each week. After each run I was to update the actual miles completed for that day. On the first training day of the new plan I dressed for an early morning run and ventured out onto the quiet peaceful streets of my neighborhood.

With my training plan set I knew the distance for each run for the next five months. It was a good feeling. My plan included four run days a week (M-T-TH-SA), cross-training on Friday, and two scheduled rest days on Sunday and Wednesday.

Figure 1 shows the last 7 weeks of the training plan. I noticed that Hal added races into his plan. He states, "One way to dispel your nervousness is to dip your toes in the water without jumping in." He went on to say that "a lot of energy is generated in the biggest [races], so you might as well get an idea of what to expect." It was good to hear Hal say that feeling nervous before a race was common (Higdon, 2016, p. 109).

Week #	Date	Mon	Tue	Wed	Thu	Fri	Sat	Sun	Total
13	8/29/22	3 Miles	3 Miles	REST	3 Miles	60m Cross	5K Race*	REST	12.1
ACTUAL									0.0
14	9/5/22	3 Miles	3 Miles	REST	3 Miles	60m Cross	9-Miles	REST	18.0
ACTUAL		3.22							0.0
15	9/12/22	3 Miles	3 Miles	REST	3 Miles	60m Cross	10-Miles	REST	19.0
ACTUAL		3.00							0.0
16	9/19/22	3 Miles	3 Miles	REST	3 Miles	60m Cross	10mi Race*	REST	19.0
ACTUAL									0.0
17	9/26/22	3 Miles	5 Miles	REST	3 Miles	60m Cross	11-Miles	REST	24.0
ACTUAL									0.0
18	10/3/22	3 Miles	5 Miles	REST	3 Miles	60m Cross	12-Miles	REST	25.0
ACTUAL									0.0
19	10/10/22	3 Miles	2 Miles	REST	3 Miles	REST	REST	CBUS-HM*	20.1
ACTUAL		2.04							0.0

* 5K Race (9/3/22) - "Pediatric Cancer 5K Pie Run"
10mi Race (9/24/22) - "Big Bad Wolfe"
13.1mi Race (10/16/22) - "Columbus Half Marathon"

Figure 1

4. My First Training Races

The 5K I signed up for in week 13 of my plan was the inaugural running of the Pediatric Cancer 5K Pie (American Pie Party, 2022). Proceeds from this race were donated to pediatric cancer research through the non-profit organization *The American Pie Party*. In an effort to draw attention to the race, the administrators included an optional whipped cream pie in the eye for any finisher who was brave enough. The field included sixty three runners of every age group from teens to sixties.

I arrived at the race location nearly an hour before the start. Those familiar butterflies were back. I set a goal to complete the race in under 30 minutes or in runner lingo, break 30 minutes, which would require a minimum 9:38 MPM. With most of my training runs in the 12-minute range, this was a stretch goal, a big stretch.

As with the Duathlon, a race organizer called the participants to attention for the playing of the National Anthem. He then instructed us that the race route included a left turn about a half mile after the start, clearly marked with a large arrow lawn sign. The race started a few moments later. As the faster runners pulled away from the main group, in only a few minutes I was running alone. As I ran, I was focused on my HR.

It wasn't long before I arrived at a main thoroughfare with a traffic light, and after the light turned green, I continued down the path. I didn't see any other runners, which should have raised a red flag in my mind. I flashed a glance at my watch and realized I had already run 1.8 miles. Then it hit me. The turn!

I immediately made a 180° turn, with my heart rate escalating more out of sheer panic than exertion. My anxious feelings were surpassed by an even greater feeling of humiliation. I eventually arrived at the turn sign, doing my best to limit walking. My very heavy breathing was a result of my elevated heart rate; so I mixed in short, 10-second stints of walking, being forced to surrender to the limits of my cardiorespiratory fitness level. As I pulled up to the finish, the race clock was approaching one hour. So much for the stretch goal.

My watch captured a total run distance of 4.85 miles for the race, meaning that I added 1.75 miles to the 3.1 mile race by missing the turn sign. I pulled out my phone and navigated to the race webpage to see my official finish time, which was 56:57. As I looked at the data, I learned that two times were listed for each participant; a clock time and a chip time. The clock time was the time of the official race clock that marked the start of the race. The chip time is initiated for each participant as they cross the timing matt at the beginning of the race. For chip-timed races, each bib number worn by each racer contains a plastic, electronic chip attached to the back side of their bib. The race timing system then captures the start and end times for each individual runner from that chip as they cross any timing matt on the course.

At the beginning of the race I chose to line up near the rear. When the race started, it took me about 10 seconds to reach the starting line. My chip time was 56:48 about 10 seconds less than my clock time, noting that it took me those 10 seconds to reach the starting matt. My chip time calculated to 18:20 MPM, measuring my time against the 3.1 mile race distance. The timing system did not know that I added 1.75 miles to the race by missing the turn.

A few days before the race I downloaded a pace app to my phone. I used this app to calculate my average MPM, using 4.85 miles as the race distance. This calculation returned an average pace of 11:45 MPM. Assuming that I would have run the race at this average pace (without missing the turn), my finish time for the 3.1 mile distance would have been 36:19 (11:45 times 3.1 miles = 36:19). This was 6 minutes slower than my 30-minute stretch goal. For the next race I decided to set a more achievable target finish time, based closer to my average pace during training. If you are wondering if I took the pie in the eye, the answer is, yes I did! Unfortunately, I don't have a photo to share.

The Big Bad Wolfe Race

After three weeks I was ready for the longest run of my life. The early hours of September 24, 2022 included a lot of rain. When I looked at the radar on my weather app, the race location was surrounded by ominous rain clouds colored in yellow, orange, and red. During my drive to the race's location, I saw elaborate bolts of lightning stretched across the sky. The rain slowed as I approached the race location and stopped when I arrived. As I parked my car there was over an hour before the start, with the intention of doing some stretches, a short warmup run, and a visit to the portable rest room if necessary. The race participation, as judged by the steady accumulation of vehicles, didn't seem to be affected by the rain. The temperature before the start was in the mid-50s Fahrenheit. The event hosted three distances, the 5K, the 10 mile, and the 20 mile. The route was the same for all distances, with the 5K turnaround at the 1.55 mile mark. The 10 and 20 mile races continued to a 5 mile turnaround, with the 20-miler going out and back twice. The pre-race butterflies were doing their thing, but less than other races. It might have been due to my preoccupation of how much rain we would have to deal with.

I had purchased a new pair of running shoes a couple of days before the race. My size for dress shoes is 8. When I bought my first pair of running shoes for the duathlon, the sales person strongly recommended I size up to 8.5 for running shoes to allow my feet room for the expansion that feet go through when running. When I bought these new shoes, the store didn't have size 8.5, but size 9 was in stock. I thought at the time that was close enough.

I set a goal finish time to break two hours. This would require that I run an average of 12:00 MPM. I based this goal on being slightly faster than my training runs leading up to the race. As the time approached for the start I saw what I believed to be some elite runners lining up near the front. I felt a tinge of anticipatory excitement at the thought of seeing what elite running looked like.

Before I knew it, we were off. At the start I felt really strong, so I pushed the pace and proceeded to pass what seemed like dozens of other runners of all ages. As was the case in the duathlon, I noticed my HR was well over 160; so I raised my hand to signal the runners behind me that I was taking a walk break. The threat of more rain passed, and the sun began to shine through partly cloudy skies. I continued my standard run-walk plan and began to feel my feet rubbing, as if my shoe laces were not tightly tied. I stopped to check and the laces were fine. It was the shoes themselves that were feeling too big. I was wearing good running socks; so I thought, *I'll figure this out after the race.* I passed the 5K turnaround and watched as the 5K runners began heading back to the start. At the 3-mile mark I slowed to a walk as I arrived at an aid station with several volunteers handing out cups of Gatorade, followed by cups of water. I took in the electrolytes and resumed my run phase.

The Elites

Maybe a half mile farther I saw in the distance what turned out to be the leader of the 10-mile race. I could hear his feet as they forcefully hit the pavement with each very fast stride. He flew past me in the opposite direction like a fast-moving train. The speed that he was running was beyond belief! Perhaps the best way to describe it is to borrow the words of Chic Anderson when he called Secretariat's record-breaking performance at the 1973 Belmont Stakes: "He's moving like a tremendous machine" (The New York Racing Association & Chic Anderson, 1973, 1:44-1:46). About ten seconds later the #2 runner passed me, running at similar speed and ferocity. Then #3, #4, and #5. As each passed me I felt a blast of wind hit me in their wake. All of them were returning to the start on the second 5-mile leg of the 10-mile run. I had not reached the halfway mark yet. I thought, *Okay, now you know what an elite, long-distance runner looks and sounds like.* I was amazed to see how any human being could run that fast.

At a scheduled doctor's appointment a few days after the race I asked my doctor if she thought a runner's heart rate was high or moderate during such an effort. She replied that generally for a runner of that caliber his heart was likely beating at a moderate pace. She added that running fast does not necessarily equal high heart rate. This was useful info for me because I noticed that my heart was progressively slowing down week after week compared to when I first started. Also my **resting heart rate** (RHR), the speed that the heart beats during sleep, was also gradually going lower. This was a good sign that my fitness was improving.

I continued on, crossed a foot bridge, just past the 4-mile mark, and then reached the 5-mile turn-around, which was clearly marked with an aid station. After receiving some much needed water I continued to the second half of the race. My feet were now aching a lot and I began regretting wearing the new shoes. The walk segments started getting longer, and the run segments were not anywhere near my starting pace. The one good thing was, I was not lost (like on the 5K pie race). This provided little solace as the heat from the bright sun started taking its toll on my energy levels.

The Finish

As my watch beeped to acknowledge the completion of mile number 9, I could see the finish area. What a beautiful site it was. I was feeling very spent. I didn't know if it was the heat, the over-sized shoes, or the fast pace at the beginning of the race. Maybe all three. As I crossed the finish line I felt lightheaded. I saw some runners sitting on a nearby curb and I moved in their direction to join them. In my depleted state I nearly fell as I sat down. Maybe it was my mind playing tricks, but the new shoes felt like I had a of couple extra inches past my toes, analogous to the giant shoes that a circus clown might wear.

I pulled out my phone and navigated over to the race website to lookup my finish time, which was 2:02:53, or 12:17 MPM. This was startlingly close to my goal considering that I nearly fainted at the finish. Then again, I had never completed a 10-mile race before. Out of curiosity I looked up the winner, a 30-year-old man who clocked a time of 53:35 (5:22 MPM). I made an association with his average pace of 5 minutes 22 seconds per mile and the speed that I saw him running toward me during the race. He seemed to be in complete control of his body as he ran and didn't show any signs of fatigue, discomfort, or pain.

Learning from Mistakes

I would be remiss if I didn't call out all the mistakes I made in this race. I call these mistakes because after the race I discovered from a number of different postings on social media that the things listed below are classic errors that have proven to be detrimental to race performance and should be avoided.

- **Never buy shoes that are not my size.** It is a big mistake to buy shoes that are not my size, either too small or too big. All the physiology that goes into running is complex enough when wearing correct-fitting shoes. If I really want to try on a particular brand and model of running shoe, and the store does not have my size, then I will ask them to order them for me.
- **Always break in new running shoes before racing in them.** After buying a new pair of running shoes, I will break them in for a couple of weeks on light training days. I will then gradually add miles or speed to those training runs before racing in those shoes. My whole body needs to get to know how the shoes feel. This includes my legs, back, and of course, feet. The last thing I need are unknown variables that new shoes bring to the heightened pressure of the race atmosphere.
- **Avoid running too fast at the beginning of a race.** Before the race starts, I will decide on a race pace and stick to it. As much as possible, I will reasonably ignore other runners and weather conditions, focusing on my pace plan for the day.
- **Avoid wearing too many layers (unless it's a winter run).** At the beginning of the race I wore three shirts to help keep me warm if it rained. Knowing the expected temperature during the race is more useful, because constant heat from

the sun depletes energy. If I feel hot, I can re-move an outer layer and tie it around my waist to allow excess heat to leave my body.

5. Inspiration from Others

During the early summer months of 2022, while I was executing my half marathon training plan I found inspiration from a few hardcore athletes. The stories of their accomplishments, especially during tough times, lifted my spirit over and over again.

The Influence of David Goggins

David Goggins served as a Navy SEAL and has been called the *"toughest man on the planet."* Within the world of extreme ultra-distance events (those that are 100 miles or more) Goggins is well known. He has completed some of the most grueling races in the world, including the Badwater 135 (run), the Moab 240 (run), and the Nachez Trace 444 (cycle). The numbers following each of these races indicates the number of miles in each race. In 2013 Goggins broke the Guiness World Record for pull-ups in a 24-hour period, completing 4,030 in 17 hours. Goggins has posted many videos on social media, encouraging people to push themselves to higher levels of inner strength. He says that when one pushes himself to his limit and he feels like he cannot go any farther, he has only used about 40% of his capacity. Goggins calls this his 40% rule, which he personally lives by. Goggins encourages people to push past mental barriers so they can find their true ability (Level Up Culture, 2022).

When I am attempting a new distance, I kept Goggins' words in the forefront of my thinking. After I completed the distance, my first thought was, *I now live in a world where I completed a [insert distance]-mile run.*

I started to choose to push through difficulties rather than surrender to them. I sensed a new confidence being built, a toughness, a tenacity. I started anticipating difficulty, even welcoming it, so that I could face it, engage it, and defeat it!

While Goggins provided me with inspiration, he is a former Navy SEAL and a lot younger than me. I wanted to find athletes pushing their limits who were closer to my age group. Well, I found two amazing athletes, Louie Ruvolo and Richard "Butch" Britton.

Louie Ruvolo

Louie Ruvolo started running ultramarathons and Ironman triathlons at the age of fifty.

When I logged onto social media, I would see posts from Louie because he and I frequented the same running groups on that platform.

In the summer of 2023 Louie submitted a post that he was anxious about competing in the Chesterfield-100, a 100-mile race. His post included his goal to complete the race in less than 24 hours. I could not fathom competing in a 100-mile race, let alone to complete it in less than 24 hours. Louie completed the 100-mile distance in 22:54:53, over an hour faster than his goal. Louie is an inspiration to me, not only for being an ultra-athlete, but because he started later in life (Ruvolo, 2018).

Richard "Butch" Britton

In Kate Champion's book *Never Too Late*, she conducts interviews with later-in-life athletes, looking to learn what motivates them and how they train. One of the athletes Kate interviewed was Richard "Butch" Britton. Kate describes Butch as a person of "pure grit and determination" who exemplifies the "deep sense of community" that is so much a part of "ultra-running communities" (Champion, 2020, p. 50).

From an early age Butch was very competitive and this spirit stayed with him into adulthood. Directly following high school, Butch served in the U.S. Marine Corps. After his discharge he entered the private sector, working in the banking industry. Following decades of sedentary living (this sounded familiar to me), he met a man at a work conference who had just completed an Ironman triathlon in Hawaii at the age of 66! This was a wake-up call for Butch (this also sounded familiar). Following this conversation with the triathlete, Butch looked at the couch and saw an indentation where he would spend a lot of his time. Butch was 56 years old and said to himself, "I can either wither away and become an old man, or I can do something about it." He started the next morning to run one mile. He said it nearly killed him (Champion, 2020, pp. 52-53).

Over the next three months he worked his way up to 3 miles. Eight months later he ran a half marathon with his niece, which he said also almost did him in. He continued adding miles to his training. He then set his next goal to complete a full marathon and shortly after that his first 50K (31 miles). Butch was never concerned about his speed—he was only interested in finishing his races. If he was able to run, he ran. If he couldn't run, then he walked. After completing the 50K Butch mentally struggled with the idea of running a 50-mile race. Finally after some years he mustered the courage and on his first try completed a 50-

miler. He asked himself, "Why had I been stressing about this for so long?" By the time Butch turned 63 he had completed 62 ultra-marathons, including a dozen 50-milers, six 100Ks, and two 100-milers (Champion, 2020, pp. 53-57).

When Kate asked Butch for his final thoughts, he advised Kate's readers to, "Please stay active. There's a mountain of evidence supporting the benefits of regular movement that includes lower cholesterol, lower blood pressure and glucose levels." Butch advises everyone to "take 30 minutes out of your day . . . go for a walk . . . and see what a difference it makes to the way you feel" (Champion, 2020, pp. 69-70).

A Sense of Community

As I took in the achievements of David Goggins, Louie Ruvolo, and Butch Britton I found myself starting to emulate the way they approached challenges. This created a type of fellowship with them, like joining the "face difficulty club." My old attitude of doubting myself was being replaced with a new attitude of testing my limits.

Goggins says in one of his videos, "Your mind quits before your body does" (Goggins, 2024). When my mind tried to convince me of a long-standing limit, I started pushing past it to see if my body could do more. For example, when the thought came to take a walk break during a run, I delayed the decision by selecting a landmark a little further down the path. I began to see a line in my life where my mind's comfort zone lived. I began stretching my comfort zone further and further.

I was becoming more aware of different degrees of difficulty and discomfort that were not injuries but a line that I had not tested or challenged yet. When I pushed past these limits I was creating a new line and at the same time training my mind that the earlier boundary was not a threat to my health and well-being. My mental limits could indeed be challenged. As I practiced doing this with small goals, my body responded positively time and time again.

Two Types of Fitness

I want to pause briefly from my running experience and cover a general understanding that I discovered about **run fitness**. I discovered a kind of paradigm of two types of fitness; **performance** (speed) and **capacity** (endurance). The level of fitness required to run fast over a short distance, like completing the 100-meter dash, is developed differently than running a further distance. It was practical for me to understand that improving my fitness level for both of these types of fitness takes time, consistency, and persistence. Improvements in my fitness are built gradually over weeks and months of consistent training.

Part of me believed that I could build fitness faster than others, or said another way, that I believed that I was in better shape than I actually was. I held this belief before signing up for the workplace fitness bootcamp (back in Chapter 1). In the words of the late Jeff Galloway, former US Olympian and running coach, "The key to goal setting is keeping your ego in check." Galloway goes on to say that an improvement of 3% to 5% is realistic (Galloway, 2016, p. 43).

After reading this from Galloway, I realized that I was expecting dramatic improvements too quickly. Immediate improvements in my race times was not only unrealistic, but it was placing my body at higher risk for injury. I decided to adjust my attitude and accept 5% as a reasonable max for improvement. This decision required humility on my part. As I submitted to this new standard I needed to remove my ego as the sole influence when setting goals for faster race times and longer race distances.

Even though my speed was improving, I was more interested in running longer and longer distances. I realized that in order to finish longer distances I would need to slow down my average running pace to conserve my energy. As my fitness gradually improved I hoped to see faster times at all the distances I was racing.

6. The Big Day Arrives!

The morning of October 16, 2022 was special for me because it marked the day I would be running my first half marathon. With my clothes and shoes prepped from the night before, I proceeded with my regular morning routine.

A Different Race Atmosphere

For this race my wife dropped me off so that I didn't need to deal with parking. I arrived at the race about an hour before the start which was at 7:30 A.M. The temperature was around 42 degrees Fahrenheit with no rain in the forecast.

Columbus combines the marathon and half marathon races on the same day with both distances starting together. All runners approach a large intersection near the end of the half marathon course. The half marathoners are directed to turn left to their finish line, while the full marathoners continue to the second half of their race.

The racing bibs are colored to quickly identify which distance each runner is registered for, orange (half) and blue (full). Columbus provides four corrals to classify the runners by their expected finish time. The fastest runners are assigned to Corral A and so on, down to Corral D, where I lined up toward the back.

A Huge Crowd of Athletes

After exiting the car I joined a group of runners who I assumed were walking toward the starting corrals. The entry area to the corrals was narrowed by temporary fencing and a large overhead banner that read, "Athletes Only Area." Everyone permitted to pass through this entrance was required to have a racing bib pinned to their clothing.

This was the first time I observed a broader use of the term athlete. Throughout my life, the term always meant a person who was strong and fast. While this is a fair definition, it is also a narrow definition. According to Merriam-Webster's Dictionary, an athlete is "a person who is trained to compete in athletics" (Merriam-Webster, 2020). If I used this definition, I would be included, along with all the other folks who spent any time training in preparation for the race. The dictionary does not place an age limit on the definition, and this race included twelve female and thirteen male age groups, from teenagers to folks in their seventies.

I began embracing the idea that the word athlete is a noun and that many different types of athletes exist. This includes world-class, professional, Olympic, college, high school, middle school, and grade school. According to the World Masters Athletics website, older adults, like me, who compete in sports are called "masters athletes," which can include any person 35 years or older (World Masters Athletics, 2025).

The United States organizes track and field sport participation through an organization called, USA Track & Field (or USATF for short). The USATF website describes their organization as the governing body for track and field sports at the Olympic, high school, and junior high school levels. The USATF also hosts running championships for masters athletes in the marathon, half marathon, 15K, 10K, 5K, and 1 mile distances (USATF, 2025). After finding the above information on competition for older adults, I began to let go of the limiting thought that I was too old to participate in sports such as running. This was a freeing experience for me.

I was mostly interested in simply finishing the race, but I also set a general time goal of breaking 3 hours. My plan was to alternate between 3 minutes running and 1 minute walking.

The Long Walk from Corral D

After the National Anthem and associated fireworks the race commenced. This included releasing the wheel-chair division five minutes before the runners in corral A (the elites). It took over fourteen minutes for my area in corral D to reach the starting line. While we slowly walked, there seemed to be an electric excitement in the air. This was not like any other race I had participated in. As I approached the start line I loaded the run app on my watch and pressed the start button as I crossed. All the nerves and excitement faded as I focused on the repeating task of 3-minute run and 1-minute walk.

During the early miles my pace was averaging between 12:00 and 13:00 MPM. I noticed a couple of ladies power-walking. I ran past them. A bit later during one of my walk breaks I saw the same two walkers pass me. As the race progressed, we repeated this alternating passing experience several more times.

Celebration and Aid Stations

As I moved through my early paces, the sheer volume of the different bands and DJs playing their songs, the screams from family members who found their racers, and all the hundreds of signs were overwhelming. This peripheral celebration did not let up as I moved through the first half of the race.

The aid stations were also a new experience as I saw many hundreds of crushed paper cups all over the street, showing the evidence that many runners and walkers had already passed through. I learned that running while trying to drink a cup of Gatorade results in more liquid splashing on my shirt than entering my mouth, so I decided to walk through the aid stations.

The Middle Race

After passing the halfway mark, 6.55 miles, I started feeling that the race would be over soon. This feeling grew stronger even though I could feel a quiet fatigue building in my legs. Around mile 9 I decided to break from my 3-minute/1-minute run-walk plan and randomly walked a little longer between some runs.

The Final Mile

As I passed the 12-mile mark a euphoria of emotions were building with each block that I completed. The other race participants in my immediate vicinity were spread very thin, which allowed me to focus more exclusively on my run/walk plan and minimize competitive impulses. My earlier leg fatigue was overshadowed by the elation of this last mile. My daughter, who was tracking my location on the race website, sent me a text message that appeared on my watch: "You're almost there! Keep going!!"

The route took us over a wide bridge in downtown Columbus and soon afterward I arrived at the junction point that I mentioned at the beginning of the chapter. As I took the turn into the finish area the crowd that was gathered there was doubly up beat—cheering loudly and flashing all kinds of encouraging signs.

I noticed some walkers about 50 feet ahead of me and then realized it was the same two that I had seen near the beginning of the race. All emotions left me for a moment as a new mini-goal of finishing ahead of them became my top priority. I turned up whatever speed I had left to pass them and created a sizable gap, so that even if I needed to walk some of the way I would still finish ahead of them. The finish line was clearly in view, a couple of blocks ahead.

As I approached the finish line my emotions got the better of me and I nearly teared up as I crossed. I caught sight of a large group of people beyond the finish line, all wearing identical red shirts. These were the medical volunteers. I caught view of one particular middle-aged gentleman on the medical team who was watching me closely with an alarmed look on his face. He obviously noticed my burst of emotions and was ready to intervene to give me aid should that be required. As I walked past him in the finish area I mentioned to him that I was ok and what he saw was pure elation at finishing the race. He did not verbally respond to me and his alarmed look remained unchanged.

After receiving my finisher medal, I was directed, along with all the other finishers, toward a long line of tables with water bottles, bananas, and other treats. *It's done!* I thought. I was so elated that I declined one of the foil wraps that volunteers were handing out to every finisher. This foil wrap creates a nice barrier from the cold wind. It was ill-advised for me to decline the wrap as it took me a fair amount of time to find my wife, while the cold wind delivered its persistent and merciless onslaught. In the future I will always accept the foil wrap when offered one after completing a race. The foil wrap can always be disposed of if not needed, but when I needed one and didn't have one I learned a hard lesson.

Taking Walk Breaks

I am pausing here to review my use of the term **finisher**. The medal one receives when completing a race is called a finisher medal. It represents the person's completing the race. It is not called a "person who ran the whole race without walking" medal.

Throughout this book I shared that I follow a run-walk training routine within the framework of the 80/20 running method. This method purposefully strives to keep 80% of my runs at a slow and easy pace. To me this means that I strive to keep my heart rate in **zone-2**, that is, no higher than 75% of my maximum heart rate. In order to accomplish this, it was necessary for me to take walk breaks on all my runs and races.

When I first started running, I held a subtle subconscious belief that if I walked any portion of a run, then I was not really a runner. In the wise words of the late Jeff Galloway, "Almost every day a new runner reports to me that an experienced runner said something like this: 'If you take walk breaks, you're not a runner.'" Mr. Galloway goes on to say, "When someone says this to me, my comeback is the following, I've been on the U.S. Olympic team and have run for more than 50 years, and I didn't know that there was a running rule book that excludes walking. Could you show me this rule book?" (Galloway, 2016, p. 19). Galloway is the author of the book *The Run-Walk-Run Method*, which teaches that walking is not only permitted during runs, but can be an essential element of building cardio-respiratory fitness.

NOTE: Jeff Galloway passed away on February 25, 2026 at the age of 80. Jeff's love for runners impacted millions of people and is best described by his lifelong friend and fellow runner Amby Burfoot, ". . . [Jeff] graduated more healthy, happy runners than any other program I have known" (Burfoot, 2026). The running world has lost one of its champions. Jeff, you will be missed.

Hal Higdon also weighs in on walking as an "excellent exercise that a lot of runners overlook in their training" (Higdon, 2016, p. 122). Hal adds, "In coaching marathon runners, I usually recommend that they walk through the aid stations to allow them to drink more" (Higdon, p. 122).

Listening to the opinions of these men was freeing to me because I needed to take walk breaks in order to lower my heart rate and perceived exertion. As I allow my body to recover during walk breaks, I am cooperating in the fitness-building process.

Distinctively New Feelings

Upon arrival at home, I went straight into a hot tub. All the muscles in my legs felt quite sore, especially my hamstrings and quadriceps. The jets firing that warm water brought me pure heaven. My wife prepared an amazing dinner for me, surf-n-turf (steak and lobster). It was the best I had ever tasted.

I learned that when I push myself in training and races I should expect a higher level of **delayed onset muscle soreness** (DOMS), which can last up to 72 hours following intense exercise (Sutton, 2022, p. 451). Experiencing DOMS is not an indication of being injured, but I did feel a higher level of soreness. I planned to rest for a day (or two). I wondered how I would feel in the morning after a good night's sleep. To my surprise, I woke refreshed, with 80% of the soreness gone.

Completing the half marathon felt like just the beginning. The half marathon was not a once-in-a-lifetime challenge. I was hooked and felt like my life as a runner was just getting started.

7. Irrational Exuberance

The week following the half marathon, I signed up for a nearby 5-mile race, called the Circleville Classic. It was a loop route that weaved through the side streets of a quiet community with the last 400-meters finishing on the local high school track. As this race started, I noticed a tall gentleman running at a very consistent pace while I continued following my run/walk plan. Toward the end of the race, this gentleman was a bit ahead of me. I sped up my cadence and slowly cruised past him. About a block later the route directed us into the high school stadium for the closing lap around the track. I finished the race with a time of 53:42, or 10:45 MPM. The tall gentleman finished exactly 2 seconds after me. After the race he mentioned to me that when I passed him he tried his best to catch me. He disclosed to me that he was 79 years old and had started running at the age of 70. He went on to tell me that the more he ran, the better he felt, and it fired up his competitive spirit too! This was amazing to me. He was 19 years older than me and he finished just 2 seconds behind me! I learned a good lesson from him. Investing in my health through daily movement improves my quality of life, no matter how old I get.

The Final Races for 2022

After having so much fun at the Circleville Classic, I decided to search for other autumn races. I found four more; the Running Scared 5K (October 29), the Dash for Camp 5K (November 12), the Hungry Turkey 10K (November 26), and the Hot Chocolate & Egg Nog 10K (December 10).

At the Running Scared 5K I met a gentleman who looked about my age or maybe a little younger. He asked me if I ran a lot, and I told him I had just started running earlier that year. He then told me he loved running and he has been running for a number of years—all 5K races. I asked him how old he was, and he told me he was 65. *Wow! I hope I look as good as he does when I'm 65!* I thought.

As we gathered at the start line, I positioned myself in the back. This route was a big loop that started and ended at the local high school. With this being my second 5K race, I decided to try running the full distance with no walk breaks. Early in the race the route crossed a side street that was open to local traffic. An elderly woman decided to drive through the race route. A young lady runner just ahead of me moved forward to try and slip past her car and was nearly hit. I saw her put her arms out and make contact with the right side of the vehicle hood. Thankfully she was not hurt and continued on. The elderly lady stopped her car so that the main body of runners could pass through.

Maybe it was the lack of walking, but I began to feel like the race was finishing quickly. Before I knew it I was on the last mile and could see the finish line. I was pushing hard at this point, huffing and puffing and just able to keep running. As I approached the finish line, I could see minute 29 ticking on the race clock. I made a final push to the end, crossing the finish with a time of 29:50 (9:36 MPM). That was wild! This time was nearly 6 minutes faster than my [extrapolated] Pie 5K time (had I not missed the turn), and I broke 30 minutes for the first time in a 5K race.

A Garmin® Smartwatch

Earlier in the year, my daughter suggested that I try some high intensity interval training (HIIT) classes from a chain gym that she was attending. HIIT is a training method that deploys periods of near maximal intensity separated by rest periods of varying lengths (Sutton, 2022, p. 32). During one of those HIIT classes I learned that some of the attendees use a Garmin watch for health tracking. One reason that these watches are popular is their capability to pull heart rate data once per second. This was very interesting to me because the main measurement I use a smartwatch for is to capture accurate heart rate data. After reviewing several different models online I decided to purchase one along with a Garmin bluetooth heart rate strap.

Once the watch was setup I discovered that Garmin designed their watches to connect to a smartphone app, called Garmin Connect®. This is an Internet-hosted system managed by Garmin to store all activity data captured by the watch. One benefit to Garmin Connect is that if the watch is damaged, lost, or stolen, all the data from the watch can be loaded onto a replacement Garmin watch. I can access the Garmin Connect system from my smartphone app or my computer web browser. Garmin also has a development environment to create custom training applications that can be downloaded to Garmin watches. These apps can be developed by anyone in the fitness community who learns the Garman development system. Some of these developers charge a fee to download their apps, but many are free. With the purchase of this watch I got the feeling I had just opened a door to a whole new universe.

The instructions on the watch for tracking a run are very straightforward. I would soon discover that my new Garmin watch had a feature called run/walk detection. This feature automatically detects when I am running or walking during an activity and separately totals all the minutes and seconds that I ran and walked. This became a very valuable metric for me that I would capture in my daily running log for every training run and race.

Boundless Enthusiasm

My experiences running the last three races of 2022 were a mixed bag of triumphs and other things.

It was a bright, sunny Saturday morning for the Dash for Camp 5K. I was fresh off my sub-30 performance a couple of weeks earlier in the Running Scared 5K. I thought to myself, *Records are meant to be broken!* I was getting used to the pre-race butterflies and actually started looking forward to them as a type of precursor to good performances.

As with my last 5K race I decided to try to complete this race without any walk breaks. I started the race at a 9:45 MPM pace and increased my speed to 9:32 MPM during the second mile. I was unable to maintain this faster pace and took a 30-second walk break during the third mile. As I took the turn toward the finish I could see the large race clock adjacent to the finish line. The time was reporting past 30 minutes; so I slowed over the last 50-meters, knowing that a new personal record (PR) time was not going to happen today.

After finishing, I looked up my time on the race website. To my amazement my chip time was 29:46, bettering my last 5K time by 4 seconds. I then recalled that the gun time for a race will always be ahead of my chip time (because I start races toward the back of all participants). Even more surprising, I discovered that I placed first among the three

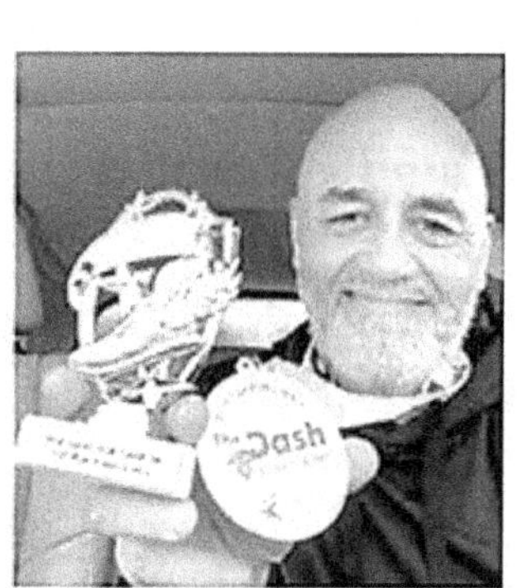

Dash for Camp 5K (11/12/22)
Photo by Bobby Schuler

runners in the male 60+ age group. This afforded me a nice little trophy that read, "The Dash for Camp 5K — 1st Place Male 60+."

The Hungry Turkey 10K was scheduled the Saturday after Thanksgiving. It was colder now, in the upper thirties Fahrenheit with some occasional snow flurries. This race was 6.2 miles, weaving through the walking paths along the Scioto River. From a goal time perspective, my thinking was, *if I was able to break 30 minutes on a 5K, why not try to break 60 minutes on this 10K?*

At the start of the race I felt very strong, but decided to keep my pace moderate in the beginning—after all, it was over 6 miles. I mixed walk breaks in when needed and kept an eye on the time with the new Garmin watch. By the halfway mark I was past 30 minutes, so I would have to pick up the pace if I had any chance of finishing under 60 minutes.

I distinctly recall arriving at the halfway point in the race where a young man was standing to mark the spot. There were four or five different paths that converged at this general area; so I asked that young man if the closest path was the path I should follow for the second half. He sleepily nodded his head; so I proceeded down the path I was pointing toward, even though I didn't see any other runners on this path. This is when all rational thought left me.

For some unknown (and irrational) reason I thought, *There's no one else here. I must be in the lead!* I continued down this path, which became more and more desolate. I thought, *This is strange. Shouldn't there be other runners following behind me?* Sticking with my earlier absurd belief of being in the lead, I continued running down this path until I arrived at a four-foot chain-link fence that abutted a major highway with cars flying at 60+ mph just inches from me. *Okay, this can't be right,* I thought. I looked around and apart from the speeding cars there was not a living soul to be seen for what looked like miles in every direction. A dreadful, sinking feeling of being completely lost waved over me and I thought to myself, *What do I do now?*

I looked down at my new watch, which showed that I had already run nearly 6 miles. I pressed one of the buttons on the watch, hoping that somehow this device could help me out of this mess. A menu appeared with options, one of them being by God's providence, *BACK TO START.* I pressed the button associated with this option and two sub-options appeared, *TracBack* or *Straight Line.* I chose TracBack and then a map and directional arrow appeared on the watch that moved as I turned the watch in different directions. The watch was directing me back to the start via GPS signaling. I began running, keeping the arrow in the 12 o'clock position, which was the implied direct route back to the race starting point. The watch retraced my steps back to the spot where I had spoken with the young man. I then realized that the race was simply out and back—and I was now officially beginning the second half of the race. The watch continued to advise me to follow the same route that I ran in the opposite direction from the first half of the race.

With about three-quarters of a mile remaining, I could see the finish line and the race administration team packing up to leave. When I arrived at the finish I stopped the run activity on the watch, which reported that I ran a total of 10.89 miles. The race timing coordinator told me that he would post an extrapolated time based on my average pace of 10:58 (had I only run the "actual" 10K distance). This was like my first 5K race where I missed the turn, except today's race was twice the distance and twice the humiliation! My actual run time for the day was 2:00:47. Ironically, I was the only male in the 60-64 age group in the race; so from an age group perspective, I finished in first place (and also last place).

On the Monday following I was on a team conference call at work and our director asked if anyone had anything interesting to share from the Thanksgiving weekend. I raised my hand and shared an abbreviated version of the above story. Suffice it to say, there were team members screaming in laughter.

The last race of the year was the Hot Chocolate & Eggnog 10K. Even though it was December, temperatures remained similar to the last race, in the upper thirties Fahrenheit with partly sunny skies. This time I made sure to confirm the race route, which was out and back. I thought, *I'm not getting lost today!* The turnout for this race was about half the number of runners in my last race. With a great sense of humility I set a sub-60 minute goal for the race in my mind.

In this race and in other races there always seemed to be a time when I found myself running alone, not because I was lost, but due to some runner "law" that seems to cause gaps to form between runners. While not having other runners around me to confirm the route, I decidedly kept a sharp eye on the direction signs in the grass for every turn, not missing any of them. I reached the turn-around, which had an "impossible to miss" orange cone in the middle of the path with a large sign that read, "10K TURN-AROUND."

On the second half I found myself running more and walking less. Glancing at my watch I could see that my time was on pace for sub-60. Within a mile of the finish there was a twist in the road on a steep downhill going out, but now a steep uphill returning. Running up that hill was brutal and I ended up walking most of it. After clearing this hill I resumed running and with only about a half mile remaining, I increased my speed to the finish. I asked a race administrator at the finish area if he could look up my time. He showed me his laptop screen which displayed my finish time of 1:00:04—missing my goal by 5 seconds!!

Initially disappointed I stopped for a moment and thought back to a month earlier, when I achieved a new 5K PR by 4 seconds. My training allowed me to run this 10K very close to 60 minutes and at the same time achieving a new PR. It was time to be grateful—both for the PR and for not getting lost again.

Part III: When Timid Becomes Tenacious

8. Taking on a Marathon

Starting in early January 2023 I reviewed my training log and discovered that I ran/walked a total of 353 miles over 107 runs and 9 races. I was feeling a nagging tightness on the outside of my left leg and knee. Thinking back, I could not pin-point the exact time when the tightness began.

I searched the Internet for "runner outside leg tightness." The search returned a condition called an **overuse** injury. It made sense to me, because I was still new to running and my body was still adapting to that much training. Another new term to me was included in these Internet results, something called Iliotibial Band Syndrome, or IT-Band Syndrome for short. *What is the IT band?* I thought.

According to Merriam-Webster, Iliotibial Band Syndrome is lateral pain outside the knee caused by inflammation through overuse, such as in long-distance running (Merriam-Webster's Medical Dictionary, 2016). As I continued investigating IT Band injuries online, I came across several videos that demonstrated strengthening exercises that were specifically intended to address the tightness and discomfort I was feeling. One of these exercises was called the invisible chair.

The invisible chair exercise involves aligning myself with my back to a wall, placing the center of my shoulder blades against the wall, and bending my knees as if sitting in a chair. This is an isometric exercise, because I was required to hold the tension on my knees for a certain number of seconds without moving any muscles during the hold. At first holding this position for 10 seconds was difficult. Over time as I continued the exercise I was able to hold the position for 60 seconds.

I checked with my doctor and she affirmed that my symptoms sounded exactly like an over-use injury of the IT Band. I described to her the exercises that I found and she agreed that I should perform them twice daily. She then insisted that I pause running until the discomfort was 100% gone. I followed her guidance and after three weeks my left leg returned to normal with no tightness or discomfort.

Early Morning Winter Runs

In the fourth week of January after completing the rehab exercises for my left IT band I started a new phase of my training. In late January, the sun was not up until 7:45 A.M.

This meant that if I was going to run before work, I would be running when it was still dark.

My neighborhood is well lit with solar-activated streetlights and lamps on nearly every home. I obtained a reflective vest to put over two or three moisture-wicking layers, depending if the temperature was above or below 40° Fahrenheit. I also bought some small clip-on lights that are charged via a standard USB cable. I placed both lights on a strap that wrapped around my chest. One light was set to solid bright white and faced forward and the other was set to flashing red on my right side. On the mornings below freezing I wore a face mask with one large opening for the eyes only. If the streets showed any snow or ice, I would run on my treadmill instead. I'm sure there are runners out there who can safely navigate through the slippery stuff, but I saw no purpose in my taking that risk.

I agree with those who say that the experience of running on a treadmill is very different from running on the street. Some folks on social media have posted that they will not run on a treadmill because the experience ruins their street running form. I have developed the opinion that treadmills have their place in training. Treadmills are softer on the joints than asphalt streets and they provide significant control over speed and incline with a high degree of precision. This is useful to me because I can choose the exact speed and incline I want. Running (or walking) up an incline on a treadmill is a useful workout for me, especially because the vast majority of the streets in my neighborhood are flat.

Returning to Running after Rehab

I understood that some of the fitness that I gained through the last 6 months of 2022 was lost during the IT band rehab period in January. Starting in February I didn't waste any time establishing a 5-day-per-week, early-morning run schedule, with run distances varying between 2 and 12 miles. I ran on 55 days between February 1 through April 30, completing a total of 269 miles.

With it still being winter, I had not given much thought toward choosing a target race for 2023. After discussing it with my family, I decided it was time to challenge myself to the marathon distance. I chose the Columbus Marathon, registering in late March, which would give me about seven months for training.

Training Paused for COVID-19

In early April I woke up one morning feeling like I had the flu. I was feverish with body aches and significant fatigue. We had some COVID-19 home test kits and mine showed positive. I contacted my doctor and she asked when I started feeling the symptoms. I told her it was that morning. That late afternoon I was reading a note from my doctor (sent through the online patient portal) recommending to start me on an anti-viral medication.

After reading her message I felt a very strange pressure on my chest combined with dizziness. I had never felt anything like that before. I was standing at my home office desk on the second floor at the time. Panic waved over me, along with the thought that this might be the beginnings of a heart attack. I calmed myself down and thought that all I needed was to lay on the couch for a bit. Being concerned that I might pass out, I held the railing and quickly moved downstairs to the living room couch. I put my head on the arm of the couch and after about 10 minutes the strange feeling passed and thankfully did not return.

In 2023, the Centers for Disease Control and Prevention (CDC) released death statistics on COVID-19 by age. The highest death percentages correlated to the 50+ age groups, see *Figure 2* (CDC, 2023). With me being 61 at the time, I accepted my doctor's recommendation to start taking an anti-viral medication that interrupted COVID-19's ability to replicate. After completing a 5-day course of the medication my symptoms were reduced and I retested negative for COVID-19.

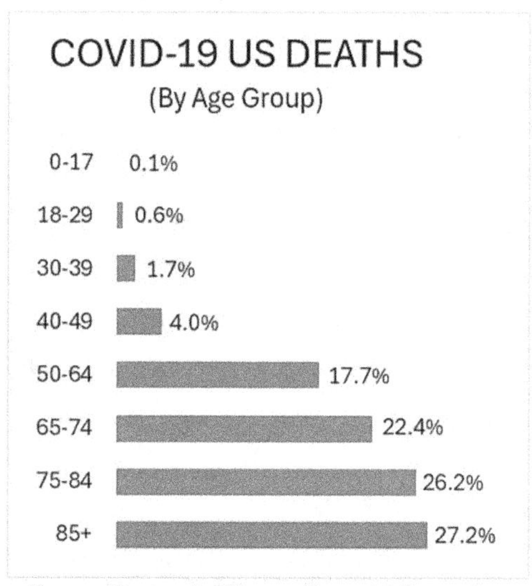

Figure 2

Peer-aged Athletes

It took me 10 days to feel recovered enough from COVID-19 to resume my training. I was regularly searching social media for other folks in their 60s who were new to running and found it as enjoyable as I did. I found several folks on social media, most of whom resided in different parts of Europe. All these folks started running in their 50s and 60s. Their exploits included completing long distance runs of 80 to 140 kilometers (50 to 90 miles). Before contracting COVID-19, I was averaging just over 35 miles per week. The races that these European runners were participating in included distances of 50K (31 miles), 100K (62 miles), and farther. This was astounding to me!

These long races are collectively referred to as ultramarathons, or ultras for short. An ultra is any race that goes beyond the standard distance of a marathon, 26.2 miles. All the European runners that I was following on social media were in their 60's and running ultra distances.

I began to think, *If I've already signed up for the Columbus Marathon, then why not consider a 50K race?* As I contemplated the decision to attempt a 50K race, a battle ensued in my mind. On the one hand I thought, *Am I ready to take on an ultra when I have not even completed a marathon yet?* On the other hand when I added all the runs and races that I had completed from August 2021 through June 2023 they totaled 830 miles. When I divided that mile total by 31 miles (i.e., a 50K race) technically I had run almost 27 50K races (in the aggregate). After a few more minutes of contemplation I settled the matter in my mind and began searching for a 50K race.

I found the Chicago Lakefront 50/50, which is an annual, dual-race event offering participants a choice of two race distances: a 50K or a 50-mile. The 2023 races were scheduled for October 28, which would allow me 12 days of recovery after completing the Columbus Marathon on October 15. I knew that an effective training plan includes a long run that approaches the target race distance. I thought, *I can use the Columbus Marathon as my last long run before the 50K race.* After signing up for the Chicago Lakefront 50K I drew a long deep breath, paused, exhaled, and said to myself, *Okay, let's build the plan.*

Creating the 50K Training Plan

I had already purchased Hal Higdon's book, *Marathon* (Higdon, 2020) for input on training for the Columbus Marathon. This book contained a training plan for a 50K race. After counting back from race day, I was left with twelve weeks.

9. Longer Training Runs

The summer of 2023 in Columbus was pretty hot and I found myself doing everything I could to avoid running in the summer sun. At this time, my doctor added a once-weekly semaglutide medication to aid in lowering my A1C, which was 6.5. In combination with all the miles I was running each week, my pant size had reduced to 32-30.

I learned to rise early, before sunrise, with my body-lights and reflective gear for many of my training runs. My running plan was filling up with completed training runs for August and September. Some of these training runs, especially on Tuesdays and Saturdays, were getting longer and longer, and I remember getting butterflies just looking at what was on the schedule the next day. A part of me felt affirmed with these apprehensive feelings because having some fear when facing a tough workout meant that I was stretching my comfort zone—which is a good thing.

A New Method

While reviewing my social media one morning a post appeared on my feed that introduced me to something called the POSE Method® of Running (PMR). After some investigation I discovered that the PMR was developed in 1977 by Dr. Nicholas Romanov. Dr. Romanov is a sports scientist who holds a Bachelor's, a Master's, and a PhD in exercise science. He received his education in Russia, the place of his birth, and relocated to the United States in 1993. The POSE Method of running incorporates some simple elements: the running pose, the use of gravity (the fall), and the pull (Romanov & Robson, 2004, p. 55-72).

The Pose, Fall, and Pull

The running pose places the body in straight alignment with one foot on the ground (support) with the knee slightly bent and the other leg lifted off the ground as if the heel of the raised leg has been pulled straight up under the hips. The lower part of the raised leg is bent at the knee and is parallel to the ground. The legs should resemble the number 4 with the support leg being the 4's vertical line and the raised leg creating the angled lines of the 4 (Romanov & Robson, 2004, p.55-60).

Once in the pose position the runner allows the body to fall forward with gravity while maintaining alignment. As the body falls forward, the ankle of the support leg bends slightly forward while the raised leg prepares to assume the support role (Romanov & Robson, 2004, p.61-66).

When using the Pose Method a runner does not reach forward with the landing foot. The landing foot simply lands under the hips in alignment with the rest of the body. Proper execution of the Pose Method ensures that the body remains in alignment because the support foot pulls up vertically. An effective mental image of the pull phase is to imagine a string attached to the back of the heel of each foot. When the raised foot lands, the string attached to the support foot is pulled vertically up, returning to the pose position (Romanov & Robson, 2004, p.67-72).

I decided to embrace the Pose Method because I discovered that this method provides me with a more efficient stride that optimizes my energy while keeping the load of my body weight in alignment under my hips. The Pose Method teaches that the runner should land on the ball of the foot, which is better equipped to accept the weight of the body than the heel or the toes. Using this method, I ran farther using the same amount of energy.

Power of the Word Only

I don't recall the day I first started doing it, but I began using the word only. I found my-self saying, "Today is only 8 miles" or "Tomor-row is only 16 miles." I found some kind of power using the word only. Some of those long training runs were the first time I ever trained at that distance. I knew I might get second thoughts on the run if my thinking was some-thing like, *Wow! I never ran this far before.* If I was going to complete a marathon and then a 50K I needed to get used to the idea that 12 miles, 15 miles, or longer runs are part of the process to get there. By saying only, I was plac-ing a type of dominance over that day's run. Also the word only added more assurance that whatever the distance was, it would be con-quered.

"Halfway" and "All of a Sudden"

Another little trick I learned was noting the halfway mark in a training run or race. I think this was berthed from the funny story of a guy deciding to swim a mile across a lake, but when he arrives at the halfway mark he thinks he can't make it; so he turns around and swims back. Instead of giving up, when I hit the halfway mark I thought to myself, *Okay Schuler, each step is worth two now!* Each step was not actually worth two; so I thought to mentally credit each second half step with the first-half step that I used to get there.

When our children were little, my wife and I would take them on many family vacation trips to the Lake Geneva area in southern Wisconsin. The drive to the resorts always seemed to take longer than the drive home. I'm not sure what this perception thing is, but it happened all the time. I applied this same concept to my arrival at the halfway mark in a run or race, planning on the second half always feeling faster than the first half.

As I approached the end of the run or race the final mile, final half-mile, final 200 meters all seemed to appear all of a sudden. I reminded myself of this, especially when the going got tough, thinking, *You'll be done before you know it.*

Energy Intake Before (and During) Runs

With the longer training runs came a new reality: expected depletion of energy. As I read more on how to improve long run endurance, the concept of fueling before (and during) long runs was a recurring topic. Many social media posts and online articles pointed me to a particular expert in the field of sports dietetics. Her name is Nancy Clark.

After a little investigation I discovered that Ms. Clark is a registered dietitian, holding under graduate and graduate degrees in sports nutrition, and the author of the best-selling book *Sports Nutrition Guidebook*.

She has advised thousands of athletes on their nutrition, covering many different sports, for high-schoolers, Olympians, and professionals. Clark states that proper fueling before and during long events can make a huge difference on how an athlete performs (Clark, 2020, p. 183).

Some athletes have reported that they refrain from eating anything before a long practice or event, for fear of gastrointestinal (GI) issues. In the case of early morning events/workouts, Clark suggests "having breakfast the night before . . . such as a bowl of cereal at 9:00 P.M. before going to bed." This way the fuel is fully digested regardless of how early the athlete is required to rise after sleep (Clark, 2020, p. 194).

After reading the above, I had no difficulty classifying myself. I'm an early riser who only takes in coffee and water before training. Fueling with light carbs the night before was appealing and it worked well for me. My new challenge was what to eat *during* a training run or race.

I saw numerous posts about energy gels and thought, *What is an energy gel?* I learned that a gel is a varied liquid paste that is sold in a pouch and provides quick energy during exercise. I searched online and found a combo pack of different flavors to give them a try. I will admit that I have a somewhat picky palate to start with; so when I tried the gels I was not surprised that the combination of texture and taste left me running in the other direction. I could not fathom how squeezing this goop into my mouth while running was going to help me; so I pressed the pause button on gels.

I decided to look in the sports section of my grocery store and found a product called honey stinger®, an energy product that contains honey sandwiched between two wafers. On the same shelf were small bags of Sport Beans®, which are jelly beans that contain electrolytes. I began taking these products during the walk portions of any run longer than 10K. The honey stingers and sport beans were terrific and caused no stomach issues during any of my runs. I decided to take half of a honey stinger (about the size of a silver dollar coin) at the beginning of each even-numbered mile of my runs. I followed this eating cadence intentionally, with the hope that the energy ingested from these products would arrive in my muscles when I ran the middle and later miles of the run.

Regarding water intake during runs, I experimented with hydration vests, waist-belts, and handheld water bottles. I tried a handheld water bottle on a couple of runs. It became evident that constantly holding the bottle created tension in the muscles of my hand. After an hour this tension became a distraction; so I decided against this method.

I enjoy using either a hydration vest or waist-belt water bottles. When using a hydration vest the device includes a vinyl bladder with a valve at the bottom that a delivery hose is attached to. When using a hydration vest, it is very useful to remove any air from the filled blatter, by holding the filled bladder upside down and using the water delivery hose to prime the water to the tip of the hose, thereby drawing all the air out of the bladder. The first time I used a vest I skipped this step and heard water sloshing in the bladder with every step I ran. A quiet water bladder, is a good water bladder. Using a vest is great for long runs or races that have limited (or no) aid stations for the runners. For shorter races (10 miles or less), I preferred using my waist-belt, which includes two 10-ounce water bottles.

In the beginning I discovered that wearing a hydration vest or a waist-belt for water took getting used to the weight of the water, especially using the vest, which held two liters of water. Using these items during practice runs was very helpful.

If a race provided aid stations with water, then I could opt to leave the vest or belt at home. It became a personal decision to judge if I preferred the convenience of having water on my person or receiving water from aid stations. I've found myself in both camps, sometimes preferring to carry and other times not to carry.

Adjustments and Extra Rest

Figure 3 shows the first 9 weeks of the 50K plan, with the actual mileage entered in the gray-colored cells. Sometimes I noticed that my body needed extra rest, which required me to make adjustments to the plan. For example, the scheduled 9-mile run on Tuesday, September 12 was shortened to 3.85-miles.

Taking an extra rest day before and/or after very long runs or races served me well. On some race days I noticed the benefit of the extra rest just before the start of the race, feeling physically and mentally fired up and ready to race. As the butterflies subsided I followed a routine of visualizing a perfectly executed race with a strong, sprinting surge at the finish.

2023 Marathon | 50K Plan

Week #	Date	Mon	Tue	Wed	Thu	Fri	Sat	Sun
1	8/7/23	3-mile run	7-mile run	Rest	4-mile run	Rower CT	15-mile run	Bike CT
ACTUAL		3.04	6.25	Rest	3.70	15 Min	15.03	33 Min
2	8/14/23	4-mile run	8-mile run	Rest	4-mile run	Bike CT	Rest	SS-15K
ACTUAL		4.02	8.03	Rest	4.02	30 Min	Rest	9.30
3	8/21/23	4-mile run	8-mile run	Rest	5-mile run	Rower CT	16-mile run	Bike CT
ACTUAL		4.12	8.07	Rest	5.25	20 Min	16.03	41 Min
4	8/28/23	4-mile run	8-mile run	Rest	5-mile run	Bike CT	12-mile run	Rest
ACTUAL		4.01	8.02	Rest	5.04	20 Min	12.02	Rest
5	9/4/23	5-mile run	9-mile run	Rest	5-mile run	Rower CT	18-mile run	Bike CT
ACTUAL		5.02	9.02	Rest	5.02	Rest	18.03	25 Min
6	9/11/23	5-mile run	9-mile run	Rest	5-mile run	Bike CT	14-mile run	Rest
ACTUAL		5.01	3.85	1.70	5.02	20 Min	14.02	Rest
7	9/18/23	5-mile run	10-mile run	Rest	4-mile run	Rest	Rest	BBW-20
ACTUAL		5.02	10.02	Rest	4.02	Rest	Rest	20.00
8	9/25/23	Rest	Rest	8-mile run	4-mile run	Rower CT	12-mile run	Rest
ACTUAL		Rest	Rest	8.08	4.03	Rest	12.02	Rest
9	10/2/23	8K base run	10K base run	Rest	5K base run	Rower CT	8-mi base run	Rest
ACTUAL		5.09	6.24	Rest	3.14	18 Min	8.02	Rest

Figure 3

The Big Bad Wolf 20-miler

It was Sunday morning, September 24, 2023. The weather was cool and dry. It was the same 5-mile course that I had run a year earlier, but this time I was running out-and-back twice to cover the required 20 miles. With completing so many first time run distances during my training plan, I felt like this was just another one. Case in point, I completed an 18-mile training run two weeks earlier while my daughter and her husband were visiting from out of town. She texted, asking if I was almost done. I replied, "Yes! I just finished the first 10. Only 8 to go" (taking full advantage of using the power of the word *only*).

As I started the 20-miler I was wearing my hydration vest, even though this race provided water stations at many mile markers. My mind was very focused on controlling the pace early on. I ran the first leg at a moderate pace, setting my watch to signal an alarm on a 4-minute run and 1-minute walk sequence. I decided to ignore what other runners were doing. I kept it very simple: just listening for my watch alarm to inform me of the next walk break. Before I knew it I took the first 5-mile turnaround, and fairly quickly I arrived at the 10-mile turnaround to begin the second half of the race. There were not many people around me because all the 5K and 10-mile participants had finished their races; only us 20-milers remained on the course.

As the race toiled on, I found myself taking longer walk breaks. I continued to remind myself that I was building new fitness with each mile I completed. Starting around the half marathon point (mile 13) my walk breaks were longer with shorter run portions. After I took the final turnaround at mile 15, I found a bit of a second wind, resuming running the majority of miles 16 and 17. My finishing time was 4:03:52, which is an average MPM of 12:12. My watch captured my average MPM pace, HR, cadence (number of strides per minute), and my average stride length (in meters) for each mile I completed in the race (*Figure 4*).

This data is useful for reviewing how my heart rate correlated to my MPM pace at different times during the race. For example, during the first four miles my heart remained in the low-140s. As the race continued, my MPM pace slowed (indicating more walking), while my average heart rate rose to the 150s. This seemed to suggest that my heart needed to recover more during the walk segments and the pace of my walking was likely too fast. I needed to learn that walking is for recovery.

With the completion of the Big Bad Wolfe 20-mile training race, the next long run on the plan would be the Columbus Marathon. All my completed training runs and races during

Big Bad Wolfe - 20-Miles   9/24/2023

Bobby Schuler (bib 502)

Miles	Avg MPM (Pace)	Avg HR	Avg P/Min Cadence	Avg Stride Length (m)
1	11:10	140	162	0.88
2	11:34	143	158	0.89
3	12:45	141	148	0.87
4	11:52	142	156	0.88
5	11:21	146	160	0.89
6	11:35	145	154	0.90
7	11:44	145	157	0.88
8	11:26	147	159	0.91
9	11:08	149	160	0.90
10	12:35	151	146	0.88
11	11:42	151	155	0.88
12	11:45	155	156	0.90
13	13:21	149	147	0.83
14	12:24	149	153	0.85
15	13:56	145	141	0.84
16	12:09	151	155	0.88
17	12:14	155	154	0.87
18	14:05	149	141	0.83
19	14:23	147	139	0.81
20	15:56	146	128	0.78

Figure 4

the early part of the training plan were part of the fitness building phase (FBP). The taper phase occurs during the final 3 weeks of the plan, before the target race. Tapering is represented by a steady decrease in weekly mileage. The taper phase allows recovery from the longest long run while bringing the body into peak fitness. Peaking is the antithesis of prepared-ness at the end of a training plan.

My training plan was a hybrid of sorts because I had two target races: the Columbus Marathon and the Chicago Lakefront 50K. I decided that my taper phase for this plan would begin before the marathon and would conclude just before the 50K race.

10. Marathon Sunday!

The date was Sunday, October 15, 2023 exactly one week following Kenyan superstar runner Kelvin Kiptum setting a new world record at the Chicago Marathon with a time of 2:00:35. The entire running world was a-buzz over how close Kiptum came to breaking the two-hour barrier in the marathon, an achievement that has never been accomplished in an officially-sanctioned race by the International governing body, World Athletics (*WorldAthletics.Org*, 2025).

By stark contrast, my thoughts were focused on finishing the Columbus Marathon. The evening prior, my wife prepared a wonderful plate of spaghetti, one of the best choices for fueling up on carbohydrates. My morning preparations were the same as always; rise early (before 4:00 A.M.), drink coffee, use the bathroom, and dress for the race. Once again I was running the longest race distance of my life.

I ordered a parking space online in advance. With the garage location loaded in my phone's GPS map app, I left the house before

6:00 A.M., thinking it wise to arrive at the parking garage as early as possible. This turned out to be providential thinking as some downtown intersections were closed off for the race and were not updated on my phone's GPS. After some anxious moments of delays in this way I finally was able to join the line of cars using the same garage.

A Sharp Poke

As I walked from the garage to the street I felt an odd, sharp poke on the right side of my right shoe, just below my ankle bone. I searched for the cause but could not find one. I continued walking and then noticed the poke again. The time was approaching 7:00 A.M., so I took a sweatband from my wrist and inserted it into my shoe to solve the problem.

The Pre-Race Build-up

I was placed in Corral C for this race because I submitted a target finish time just under five hours. My familiar butterflies transformed into excitement. I called to mind all the training in the plan and the training taper over the last three weeks. I reminded myself, *Schuler, you followed your plan. You're ready for this race.*

I arrived at the entrance to Corral C and found a spot to wait for the race to start. Today the color of my racing bib was blue, signifying that I was running the full marathon. Nearby I overheard what appeared to be some thirty-somethings talking about how nervous they were. They were all wearing orange-colored bibs (i.e., half marathoners). I decided to break the ice and ask them if this was their first half marathon. They all nodded. I mentioned to them that I had run the half last year and I went too fast at the beginning, encouraging them to take their time in the early miles of their race. I then reassured them that they would do great! Judging by their smiling response, my words seemed to settle their nerves a bit.

With characteristic flare and pomp the announcer counted down the seconds and after a burst of fireworks he blasted the start horn and the race was officially underway. From where I was standing Corral C seemed significantly closer to the start than Corral D from last year. However, we were still required to walk about three blocks to arrive at the starting line. I would later find out that this walk took nearly 13 minutes (per the difference between the gun time and my chip time).

The Start

As I crossed the start line, I felt unusually loose and strong. I found myself weaving through and passing several runners of all ages. I did not like running inside tight groups, mainly because I knew I would be taking walk breaks; so as soon as I found an open area I settled into my first-half pace. As expected, the same celebratory atmosphere of loud bands and DJs from the 2022 half marathon were present. I noticed less of the entertainment this time, choosing to focus on my pacing plan.

Around the 5K point I glanced down and noticed that the wrist sweatband was no longer in my right shoe. I again could feel the poke; so I pulled off the course and tucked one of my running gloves inside my shoe with the fingers of the glove sitting underneath my foot and the rest of the glove resting between my ankle and the inside of the shoe. That glove stayed in my shoe for the remainder of the race.

You might be wondering, why is he sharing these details about this poke in his shoe? The reason is problems happen. At such times it is most productive to seek solutions to the problems rather than complain or wonder, *Why me?* After encountering several odd little problems like this during training runs and races, I stopped questioning why these things happen. I learned that taking time to wonder why a problem happened was unproductive, especially during a race. A much better use of my time was to direct my attention to solving the problem as quickly as possible.

Bathroom Break

During mile 7, my enlarged prostate was insisting that I empty my bladder, like a persistent toddler pulling on his dad's pants to pick him up—Dad? DAD? DAAAAD! As I looked at the long lines of people waiting for a portable rest room at the current aid station I decided to hold it until the next station. Just after crossing the mile 9 marker, the request changed to an all-out imperative. Thankfully the lines were shorter and I was able to complete the urgent task quickly.

Starting the Second Half

As I watched the half marathoners enter their finish area, I glanced at my watch to see the elapsed time at 2:35, which was about 15 minutes faster than last year's half marathon time of 2:50. I had the sinking feeling that I ran the first half too quickly AGAIN! The advice I gave to the thirty-somethings before the race came to mind, with a tinge of hypocrisy. I needed to practice what I preach. Feeling a fair amount of general fatigue, I decided to walk the last quarter of mile 13.

During my walk a young man pulled up and joined me. He asked me how it was going. I told him that I ran the first half too fast and needed to walk for a bit. He proceeded to share that he was twenty-one, that this was his first marathon, that he hardly trained at all for it, and he was feeling great. I didn't mention to him that I was nearly three times his age and that this was also my first marathon. We wished each other well and he proceeded to resume a very smooth, almost gliding stride up the street, around the next turn, and out of my sight. Ah, the wonders of youth!

After taking in some electrolytes at the next aid station I felt a bit better. The course route took us into the Ohio State University district where I saw various participants moving at a similar pace as me, with some walking and others slowly jogging. It was nice to see folks around my same fitness level.

THE WALL!

As I completed a walk segment after passing the marker for mile 18, I attempted to resume a slow run. I tried to lift either leg but neither would obey. I may have even audibly told my legs to run but they would not respond. I didn't have enough energy in my legs to run or even jog! I thought, *So this must be the wall that I heard so many speak about.*

The wall (also commonly called, bonking), is the point at which a combination of energy depletion and excessive fatigue renders a runner with reduced ability to perform. It was a first for me. I didn't feel pain, just no ability to run. Each time I tried to resume running my quad muscles had insufficient energy for the task. I was, however, able to walk; so I walked from mile 18 through mile 22.

A Friendly Face

Mile 22 ended at the bottom of a hilled-street lined with single-family homes. Walking down a hill was hard on my leg muscles; so I shortened my stride as much as I could to avoid going too fast and straining my already depleted leg muscles.

Near the bottom of the hill, where mile 22 concluded, was the home of colleague from work who was also a marathon runner. He completed a 100-mile race a couple months earlier. As I walked down the hill he caught sight of me and ran up to greet me. He asked me how I was doing. I told him I had hit the wall back on mile 18 and that I was not able to run. He asked me what I was going to do. I told him I will walk the rest if I have to. He had a table setup in front of his home; so I enjoyed some of the carb-rich food and drink he had prepared and then pressed on. Seeing a friendly face was uplifting as I pressed through my fatigue.

As I continued, a jogging man-woman couple decided to join me for a walk break. I asked them if this was their first marathon. The man replied, "Oh no. This is my ninth." I smiled brightly and told him that was amazing. They didn't seem to be in the same depleted state I was in, but they were not moving too fast either. After a short conversation they resumed their earlier run and I did not join them. I picked up my walk pace and found a minimal ability to jog. I switched between jogging and walking about every 20 paces.

Completing miles 23, 24, and 25 seemed to take forever. No matter how slow I ran, it was faster than walking. I just needed my quads to agree to end their strike and join the rest of me in the remainder of the race. With mile 26 in sight I completed two of three 90-degree street turns before the turn into the finish. As I headed into the final turn, I looked at my watch, which showed 5:50 elapsed time since the start. I thought, *Wow! It took me 2 hours 35 minutes to complete the first half and about 3 hours 30 minutes to complete the second half.*

While I was pondering this, I headed into that last turn and could see the finish line a few blocks up the street. In the background of my view I saw a giant, elevated video screen in the finish area. The size had to be 40 feet in diameter and it was filled with the letters, BOBBY SCHULER. Then I heard a man say over a loud speaker, "And here comes Bobby Schuler!" I felt a wave of mixed emotions and then heard cheering from the few hundred remaining spectators! They were cheering for me? They didn't seem to notice, or care, that I was walking. I thought, *Okay Schuler, let's try to find some energy to run.* I gingerly started to jog and didn't stop until I crossed the finish line. The support team immediately placed the finisher medal around my neck and gave me a foil wrap, which I gladly received. My official finish time was 6:05:19.

The finish area was identical to what I remembered from the half marathon the year before, except this time I was on the marathon side of the street. One of the volunteers gave me a plastic bag and I began filling it with what remained of the treats prepared for all the finishers, including my favorite, a pint of cold chocolate milk. I delayed eating any of the food as I hobbled through the area marked Athletes

Only, with the sole intention of not stopping until I reached my car.

Only after climbing three flights of stairs and not finding my car did I realize that my vehicle was parked in the adjacent garage a block further up the street. I proceeded to walk back down the three flights of stairs, a block to the other garage, and back up another three flights of stairs. This extra walking turned out to be a blessing in disguise because it allowed my leg muscles to slowly loosen up after the race. It was possible that had I not allowed my muscles to cool down in this way my legs might have tightened or locked up on me.

Once in the car I began taking in some of the nutrition in the bag, starting with that choc-olate milk! Being one of the last people to finish the race, the garage was nearly empty of cars; so my departure was without delay.

Upon arrival at home I headed straight to the hot tub again, just as I did after the half marathon. Climbing the stairs was challeng-ing. I recall thinking, *I never felt like this before!* I also never hit the wall in a race before.

Most Important Takeaway

I now knew personally what hitting the wall felt like. Not fun. After downloading the mile pace numbers I observed the effect that hitting the wall had on my race time. *Figure 5* displays my mile split times for the whole race. I circled my MPM times from mile 18 to the finish, which marks the time that I first encountered the wall and where I walked most of the remainder of the race. The most important things I learned from hitting the wall was my need to understand how fuel my body and face significant fatigue during long runs.

Columbus Marathon 10/15/2023

Bobby Schuler (Bib 3006)

Mile #	Avg MPM (Pace)	Avg HR	Avg P/Mile Cadence	Avg Stride Length (m)
1	11:15	140	154	0.95
2	11:19	144	155	0.92
3	11:14	145	157	0.92
4	12:03	144	148	0.93
5	11:38	148	149	0.93
6	12:02	148	144	0.93
7	14:02	145	131	0.9
8	11:46	148	150	0.9
9	11:49	149	153	0.89
10	11:36	153	154	0.91
11	12:18	150	149	0.89
12	12:50	149	147	0.85
13	11:28	154	156	0.91
14	12:56	152	145	0.88
15	15:10	143	130	0.83
16	13:24	145	144	0.85
17	13:56	144	141	0.83
18	15:41	140	131	0.78
19	16:59	135	126	0.76
20	15:25	138	134	0.79
21	16:32	134	128	0.76
22	16:37	132	126	0.78
23	17:01	131	123	0.78
24	17:08	130	124	0.77
25	16:20	127	127	0.79
26	15:48	132	129	0.82
26.2	15:20	134	132	0.83

Figure 5

11. A Cold, Dark Morning in Chicago

The Chicago Lakefront 50/50 ultramarathon events are set on the Chicago Lakefront Trail (CLT), a mostly paved running and cycling path that stretches 18.5 miles along the scenic western shores of Lake Michigan. My race, the 50K, is an out-and-back route starting at the Foster Avenue boat house, running south to the North Avenue beach turnaround, then returning to the Foster Avenue start. This totals two 5.18 mile legs and one 10.36 mile lap. Participants repeat this route for two more laps to complete the 50K distance.

The CLT consists of two (or at times four) north/south lanes, with runners on the outer lanes and bikes inside. The race administrators made it clear to us that the 50/50 race does not have exclusive rights to the CLT on race day, so we should be mindful that non-race cyclists and runners will be present on the CLT during the races.

Conditions Before the Race

I felt physically great the morning of the race despite the cold, damp, and misty morning on Chicago's lakefront. The temperature was in the upper-30s Fahrenheit with mostly cloudy skies.

My training since the Columbus Marathon was purposely light, taking five of the twelve days for full rest. The registered participant list for the 50K was just over 100 and for the 50-miler less than forty. This was not like the huge crowds at the Columbus Marathon. My daughter and her boy-friend agreed to support me at Foster Avenue and my son and his girl-friend agreed to help at the North Avenue turnaround.

I noticed that the back windows of many of the participant cars had decals of large two-digit (and some three-digit) numbers, declaring the ultramarathon exploits of their drivers. These were very serious athletes and I felt honored to be running in the same race with them.

The Start

The 50-milers were released at 7:00 A.M. to provide them an extra hour of daylight, with an 11-hour cap on their race. The 50K race began at 8:00 A.M. with a 9-hour cap. With great anticipation to get going, I lined up in the front of the pack, something I had not ever done before. After the National Anthem played, the race commenced.

Pretty quickly I found myself in the middle of a pack running at an 8:00 MPM pace. I was not prepared to go out this fast and started to look around for a way out of the pack, but I found none. I remained in the pack for 12 minutes. When I finally got out, I took an immediate walk break, thinking to myself, *That was not how I wanted to start this one.*

I continued down the path and after several bends and turns arrived at the North Avenue beach turnaround and aid station. The timing matt was clearly marked, which each runner is required to cross before continuing on the second leg. I was feeling pretty good after this first leg, with a mostly full hydration vest of water and some honey stingers. After crossing the timing matt I decided to continue without stopping at the aid station.

I ran leg 2 with a 50/50 mix of running and walking, noting in my mind the exact landmarks but facing north this time. A group of us ran past a crowd of pedestrians enjoying the cool, cloudy morning. One of them looked at us with a big smile and asked, "How far is your race?" None of the racers ahead of me responded to her; so as I passed her I said, "31 miles." She smiled again as she shook her head in disbelief.

After Lap One (10 Miles)

As I approached the aid station at Foster Avenue at the end of leg 2, I was feeling pretty depleted. During the Columbus Marathon, I saw some people applying a roll-on instant muscle relaxer to their leg muscles; so I bought some before the race to have on hand if needed. My daughter's boyfriend was present when I arrived at the Foster Avenue aid station. He asked me if I needed anything and I asked him to pass me the roll-on. I proceeded to apply four lines to each of my quads. I could feel it working quickly. I made a stop in the portable rest room and then started leg 3.

The Breakdown Starts

It wasn't long, maybe around mile 11, that I realized I had applied too much roll-on. My quads were burning. At the same time I began feeling an odd pulling on the outside of both knees. I took a walk break, but the pull feeling continued, even when I was walking. I resumed running and the intensity of the pulling rose and dropped, like the 3 to 5-foot waves hitting the breakers on the lake. As if things weren't challenging enough, I began feeling a sharp persistent pain driving up the center of my right heel with every step, whether I was running or walking. This was, as best I could ascertain, plantar fasciitis. The pain level in my heel was high enough to overshadow the burning of my quads. Every step felt like a nail driving up into my heel. My natural reaction was to avoid any heel contact on my right foot.

I was about halfway through mile 13, when I thought, *I might be able to push through this if I was closer to the end of the race, but I'm less than halfway.* I pulled out my phone and called my daughter. My call went straight to voicemail. I called my son at the North Avenue aid station. He answered and I told him what I was facing. He told me to continue down the route and he would meet me near the aid station. I could only walk at this point, with my knee pain being masked by the more intense pain coming from my right heel.

As I continued south on the path I could see the sand of the North Avenue Beach, so I knew I was getting close to the aid station. About a block and a half ahead of me, without the aid of my glasses, I saw a blurry image of a man trying to control two big dogs. My immediate thought was, *I hope those dogs don't jump on me.* As I got closer I realized it was my son. His boxers, Bella (female) and Cooper (male) weighed about 85 pounds each and were a lot to handle. My son fitted them with two industrial harnesses that were hooked together on one military-grade leash. He was holding them with all his might in the middle of that leash. The dogs were extra-excited to be by the lake and even more so when they saw other dogs with their owners on the path.

As I got closer to them, both dogs recognized me and surged to greet me–Bella hitting me first and nearly knocking me over. My son greeted me and suggested that I continue through the leg 3 timing matt to get credit for going this far. I complied and then walked over to his car.

The dogs were already in the back seat, having changed their excited demeanor to calm cuddling. When I entered the backseat, the dogs made room for me, then proceeded to lay on me, giving me their warmth and looking at me with a settled, canine form of concern. They seemed to say with their eyes, *Hey Gramps, are you okay?* My son pulled a blanket from the back and the two dogs and me began to warm up nicely. When we arrived at the Foster Avenue aid station in my broken-down state I didn't have the wherewithal to exit the car to notify the administrators that I was withdrawing from the race (along with turning in my ankle timing bracelet) so my son did it for me.

This was my first time experiencing a Did-Not-Finish (DNF) for a race. While I was disappointed, I started to think of the things I could have done better to prepare for the race. One ill-advised thing that seemed glaringly obvious was starting in the front with faster racers and getting stuck in their pack. Another was working from a short training plan of only twelve weeks when Hal's plan spanned twenty-six. But I wasn't giving up on the 50K distance. I resolved to continue learning everything I could about ultramarathon preparation and race management, both before and during the race.

A few days after my 50K attempt, I e-mailed one of the race administrators, letting him know that I had completed my first marathon thirteen days before the 50K race. He replied to my e-mail saying, "It would have been quite a feat to run your first marathon and then turn right around and complete your first ultra! My hat goes off to you for trying." I replied thanking him for his comments and letting him know that I intended to return next year to complete the 50K race.

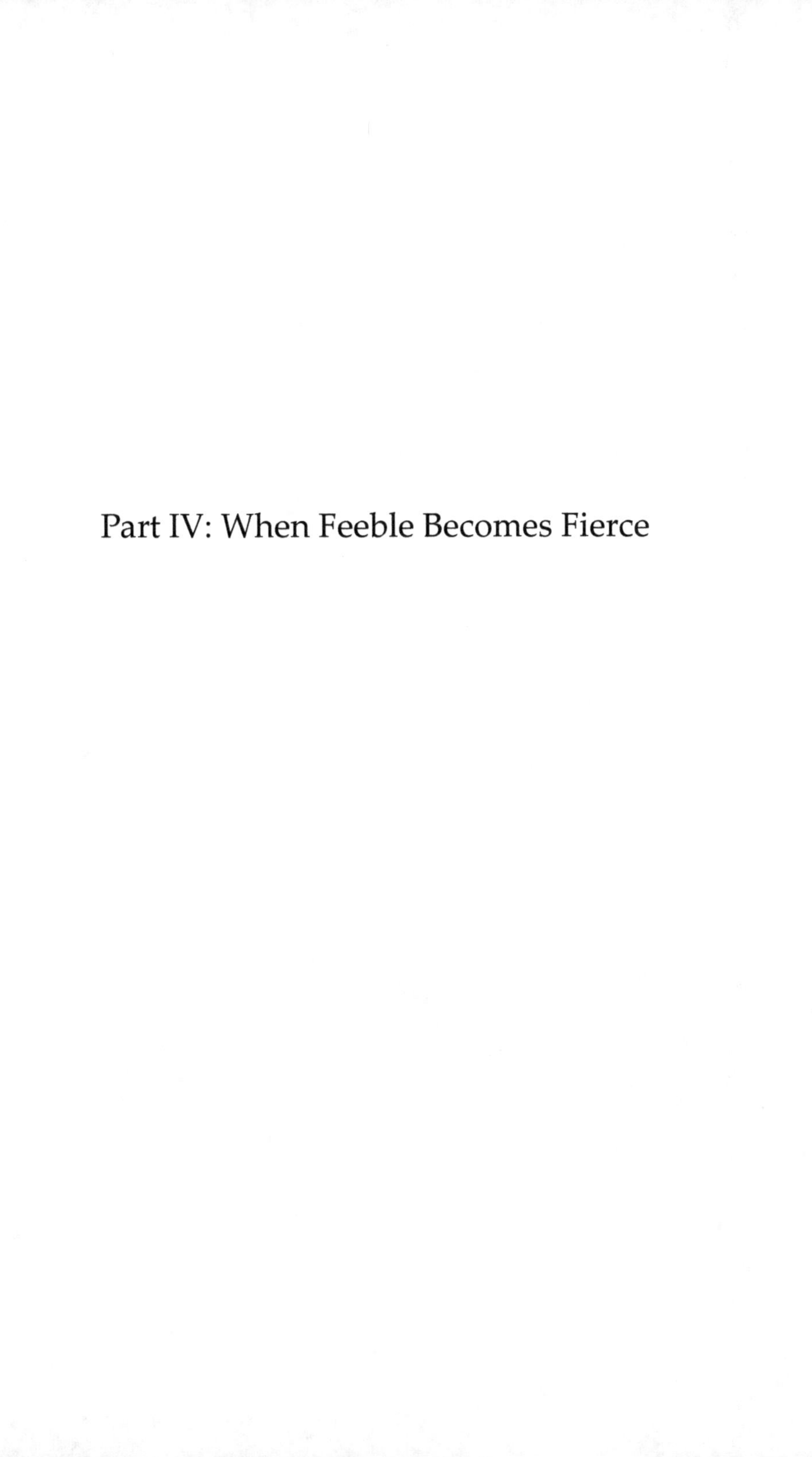

Part IV: When Feeble Becomes Fierce

12. Strength Training

In November 2023 I was shopping in my local grocery store and I noticed a tall, thirty-something young man wearing a T-shirt with the message Arnold 5K Pump & Run® printed in large letters. I asked him if he competed in the event and he affirmed that he did. I told him that I recently heard about the competition and was considering signing up. He enthusiastically encouraged me to do so telling me that I would love it.

Back home I decided to research the competition in more detail, discovering that the Arnold 5K Pump & Run (5KPR) is one of the many events associated with the Arnold Sports Festival®, hosted by Arnold Schwarzenegger in Columbus, Ohio every year in March. Columbus is an important city to Mr. Schwarzenegger because it is where he won his first Mr. World contest in 1970 (Schwarzenegger, 2026).

The 5KPR is a dual-phase event where each participant performs a bench press lift segment up to a maximum of 30 repetitions. When all participants have completed the lift segment, the competition moves to the street to complete a 5K run. For every successful lift 30 seconds is subtracted from that participant's 5K finishing time, reducing the run time by a maximum of 15 minutes. The event is designed to reward those with strength and cardio fitness by lifting the maximum (30 reps) and completing a fast 5K race. The winner is the one with the lowest adjusted 5K time (after the lift calculation is applied). The calculation for the lift portion is based on age group and percentage of body weight. Any man under 40 lifts 100% of his body weight, men in their 40s lift 90%, 50s — 80%, 60s — 70%, and 70+ lifts 60%. At that time I was 61 and weighed 167 pounds; so 70% of that amount is 116.9 pounds. When rounded to the nearest 5-pound increment my assigned lift amount for the bench press is 115 pounds (Schwarzenegger, 2026).

My Background in Strength Training

When I was 30 (a bit over 30 years earlier) a very good family friend, Victor Santiago, took the time to teach me lifting principles. Victor spent years training with free weights and it showed in his muscular physique. Victor was trained under champion bodybuilder, Mario Nieves. Victor was meticulous about me lifting with proper form so I would receive the full benefit from lifting and avoid injury. Victor directed me to exercises that covered all the major muscle groups in my chest, arms, legs, back, and core.

I remember our first lifting session very well because after the workout I was feeling fantastic. I asked Victor, "Do you really think I will feel sore tomorrow because I'm feeling really great right now?" Victor responded with a slow smile, and moving his face closer to mine, he slowly said, "Guaranteed!" The following morning, I woke up and could barely get out of bed. Every part of my body was sore! I called Victor and let him know how right he was. He told me that the best thing for me was to rest that day and then get back to the gym for another workout.

I continued strength training workouts with Victor for a few more months. Over time our busy work and family commitments made scheduling workouts together increasingly difficult. As a result, strength training slowly evaporated out of my life.

Body-Weight Training

Throughout 2023 I had been regularly performing push-ups and dips. On February 14 (Valentine's Day) I decided to try a one-hour push-up challenge. I chose to start with an up/down 1x4x1+1 pyramid (17 reps total) executed every minute. A pyramid is a progressive pattern for counting repetitions in an exercise. For example, a 1x3 pyramid involves performing 1 rep, then 2 reps, then 3 reps, for a total of 6 push-ups. This represents an up-only pyramid. When performing an up/down 1x4x1 pyramid the repetitions are counted as 1 rep, 2 reps, 3 reps, 4 reps and back down with 3 reps, 2 reps, and 1 rep, for a total of 16 repetitions. It's really just a different way of counting. I preferred using the pyramid because it gave my mind something to concentrate on while I was executing the challenge.

Each pyramid set took about 30 seconds to complete, with rest allocated to the remaining seconds in each minute. During the push-up challenge I decided to lower the repetition count to a 1x3x1+1 pyramid (10 reps total), which took me about 20 seconds per set and provided me 40 seconds recovery time after each set. I ended up completing 520 push-ups in that hour. It was both fun and exhilarating.

Resuming the Bench Press at 61

I was very curious to know what 115 pounds felt like relative to my current strength level; so I drove over to a local gym about a mile from my home and signed up for the "cancel anytime" monthly program. The next day I arrived at the gym early in the morning and walked straight over to an available bench. I loaded 35 pounds on each side of the standard 45 pound bar and took my position on the bench. After lifting 115 pounds five times, the bar felt heavy—*VERY HEAVY*. I put the bar down and realized that if I was going to successfully lift 115 pounds thirty times I would need to add strength training to my weekly routine.

I started showing up at that gym three days a week. I initially lowered the weight to 70 pounds so I could complete four sets of ten repetitions per set without experiencing total muscle failure (TMF). TMF is when the muscles performing the concentric (push from the chest) phase of the bench press exercise are depleted of energy and unable to complete that repetition (hence the word failure). In this context the word failure is not a bad thing. It is good to bring the muscles close to TMF because this is a sign that you are utilizing everything that the muscle can perform. Following the workout it is best to allow that muscle group to rest and recover for twenty-four to forty-eight hours, allowing time for the muscle fibers to rebuild stronger. Adding supplementary protein to my diet helped with this rebuilding process. I will cover more on protein in chapter 13.

Using a Spotter

It is a common practice to lift with another person who is watching and ready to help if the lifter approaches TMF. This extra person is called a spotter. Sometimes all that is needed from a spotter is a couple of fingers to help the lifter complete a difficult rep. I didn't have a spotter at that gym; so if I sensed my muscles getting close to TMF I would put the weight down, allow my muscles to recover for up to 30 seconds, and then complete the remaining reps in that set.

Challenges to Using a Public Gym

As I continued attending that gym, I discovered that it was increasingly difficult to get bench time with many other people using the benches. I inquired online to find out how much a bench, bar, and set of weights cost. I found a reasonably priced setup and ordered it online. Once my home bench was setup I canceled the gym membership and began enjoying the convenience of lifting in the comfort of my home.

Starting in December 2023 I gradually began adding equipment to my home gym. I bought dumbbells of various weights, exercise bands of various thicknesses, a chin-up/pull-up station, and appropriate racks for the equipment.

My Focus on Upper-body Muscle Groups

With the competition only about 4 months away, I knew I had a bunch of work to do to have any chance at all of lifting 115-pounds 30 times. I focused 80% of my lifting time on the bench press and the other 20% on training with dumbbells to perform other upper-body exercises, like curls, reverse curls, and butterflies. My training load included 4 sets of 10 reps per exercise, just as Victor taught me. Being the inquisitive investigator that I am, I researched online to see if there were other load methods to accelerate my strength development.

Muscle Strength vs. Muscle Size

During this time I learned a couple of new terms, progressive overload (PO) and muscle hypertrophy (MH). PO is the process of systematically lifting more weight and/or volume that triggers the body to adapt to greater loads being placed upon it, resulting in greater strength. MH is the increase in individual muscle fibers resulting in larger-sized muscles (Sutton, 2022, p. 610, 616).

What I needed was the ability to lift 115 pounds 30-times regardless of the size of my muscles. I discovered that lifting heavier weight with lower rep counts enabled me to gradually build more muscle force than lifting a moderate amount of weight with higher rep counts.

A *VERY IMPORANT* WORD ON SAFETY

While lifting in my home gym, a couple of times I brought my muscles extremely close to TMF. On one of those occasions I experienced TMF in the middle of a rep. I lowered the bar to my chest, tilted one end of the bar to the floor, and used both arms to raise the bar enough to move myself out from underneath the weight. Not a fun experience at all! On another occasion I managed to complete the repetition just as all the energy in my arms was depleted and the bar slammed down on its resting station. Equally not fun! I am *immensely grateful* that I was not injured on either of these occasions; however, these experiences brought home the understanding that my lifting setup was not safe enough!

Immediate Steps to Improve Safety

After experiencing the above TMF close calls I decided to search the Internet for a lifting system that included a mechanism for me to be my own spotter, also called self-spotting, thus being able to spot myself without having another human to act as my spotter. My answer was found in the smith machine.

A smith machine is a lifting station that has two vertical steel columns connected with hook openings in the columns at regular intervals. The lifting bar is secured through two other vertical columns, with hooks attached to the bar that insert into the hook openings.

A good quality smith machine includes stoppers that hook into the vertical openings to enable the lifter to lower the bar and exit the exercise if TMF occurs. After my smith machine was installed, I experienced TMF a few times and each time I was able to hook the bar safely without the fear of being injured. When I lift a very heavy weight, I *always* set the independent stoppers above the level of my chest to ensure my safety if the weight proves to be too heavy for me.

I feel a smith machine is a great alternative if a human spotter is not available. Safety always comes first!

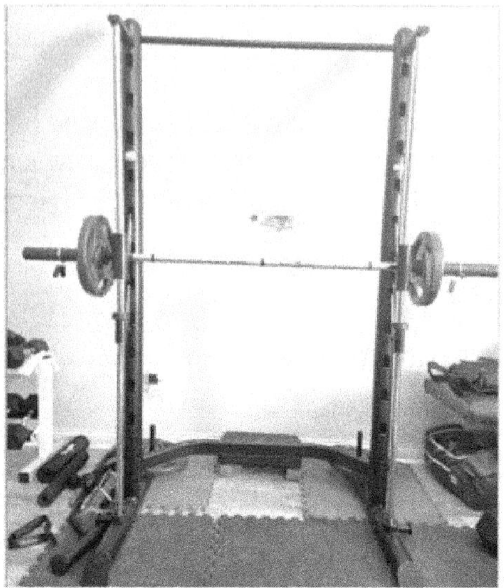

Smith Machine - Photo by Bobby Schuler

Confirming Form and Balance

While I felt that my strength training was going well, in the back of my mind I knew that I was focusing on my upper body, and not working all the other muscle groups (as Victor instructed me). I wondered if a smartphone app was out there that provided both a balanced lifting routine and training videos to remind me of proper form. In August 2023 I found an app that was not far from my original motivation for lifting in the first place.

13. Seeking Balance

My app search led me to the Pump Club® (PC) app. Who designed the Pump Club app? Arnold Schwarzenegger. Arnold personally designed all the programs in the PC app so it provides exercises for muscle growth and increased strength. The plans in the PC app are flexibly designed around the exercise modes of free weights (barbells and dumbbells), exercise machines, or body weight only (Schwarzenegger, 2023). The PC app also contains short video demonstrations of correct form for every exercise in the app. These video guides show each user the correct form for performing each lift safely and effectively (Schwarzenegger, 2023).

One of the first things I noticed about the PC app was the statement of vision that I was guided to complete during the initial setup. This was good for two reasons: (1) Arnold and his team firmly believe that writing down goals places a person at a higher probability of achieving the goal, and (2) The PC app is designed to guide the user to the training plan that best fits his or her goals (Schwarzenegger, 2023). Writing down my goal was pretty simple: to be able to perform the bench press 30 times using 115 pounds.

Training the Whole Body

Once I started using the PC app, the training plan I selected was geared toward increasing my strength. Starting the first day, I quickly discovered how much I was ignoring the major muscle groups in my legs, back, and core. The PC app guided me through a balanced workout that covered all the major muscle groups. The workouts in the app gave attention to every detail in a workout, including providing a count-down timer to ensure the lifter is getting sufficient rest between sets and exercises. This was appealing to me because previously I was not always consistent in providing my body with sufficient rest between sets.

Some of the workouts included combination exercises, also referred to as a superset or triset. A superset is the combination of two different exercises performed back to back with little or no rest in between. The reasoning behind a superset is to create an adaptation that the body is not accustomed to and thereby stimulate new growth and strength. A triset adds a third exercise, executed in the same way as a superset. Supersets and trisets are commonly designed to focus on a single muscle group from two or three different movements or directions (Schwarzenegger, 2023).

As I began performing leg exercises, such as squats and deadlifts, a fascinating thing happened. My runs became easier. Previous to beginning strength training, I thought my legs were getting sufficient attention from all the running I was doing. This was partially correct. I can't recall how many social media posts I read that speak about the weekly training habits of elite runners that included various types of strength workouts. I am not an elite runner, but I wanted to improve my running form and the strength of all the muscles I use when running.

The Role of Amino Acids and Protein

As a part of subscribing to the PC app, members receive multiple training e-mails from Arnold and his team. These e-mails are filled with a wide variety of research articles on fitness, nutrition, and many other health topics. The subject of protein is a topic that receives good attention in these e-mails.

Protein is the macro-nutrient that feeds muscle development and growth. Proteins are made up of long chain amino acids. The human body requires 20 amino acids with 9 being essential and only acquired from the food we eat. Regardless if someone desires to grow muscle size (hypertrophy) or muscle force production (strength), protein is the macronutrient that fuels that effort (Wolfe et al., 2008).

Volumes of books have been written on protein. The term **sarcopenia** speaks to age-related decline of muscle tissue. **Metabolic aging** is the rate of decline in overall metabolism relative to a person's chronological age. Both sarcopenia and metabolic aging are concepts that shine a light on the importance of daily protein intake in the diet of adults 50 years and older. The adult recommended dietary allowance (RDA) of protein is 0.8 grams per kilogram of body weight. Research has shown that this level of protein intake is not sufficient for older adults to maintain their health. This is because the aging process causes up to 5% loss in muscle mass each decade, starting at age 30. With this added muscle tissue decline, older adults should increase their daily protein intake to 1.0 to 1.5 grams per kilogram of body weight (Wolfe et al., 2008).

In late 2023 I began protein supplementation in the form of protein shakes. With the combination of lifting and increased protein intake, I started to see both muscular growth and strength increase throughout my body. Carrying a 5 gallon bottle of water to the home dispenser was no longer an intimidating task. I welcomed my increased strength not only because I could do more, but because I no longer felt the muscle aches and pains caused by so many years of low activity.

Part V: When Hidden Becomes Revealed

14. More Health Challenges

In the beginning of 2024 my training schedule was quite rigorous. I was preparing for the 2024 5K Pump and Run competition that was scheduled for March 3. During the first three weeks of February I shifted to more lifting and pulled back on my running, logging 16 run days and 11 heavy lifting sessions. What I didn't know was the Norovirus was spreading through our area and was about to hit me like a ton of bricks.

Norovirus in Late February

Norovirus is a flu infection. As defined by the Cleveland Clinic, norovirus symptoms include "nausea, vomiting, watery diarrhea, and painful stomach cramps." I battled the infection most of the night of February 22 and was completely drained of energy the following day. The core infection from norovirus is rooted by influenza, a respiratory virus, according to the Cleveland Clinic. Within two days, I was coughing constantly as the virus settled in my lungs (Cleveland Clinic, 2023).

While I fought the norovirus symptoms I was unable to run or lift for the rest of February. I continued coughing right up to the day of the 5K Pump and Run competition. A debate raged in my mind, *Do I show up or do I not show up?* I decided to skip the competition, knowing that I would push myself hard, especially during the 5K run, which would adversely affect my recovery time.

When It Rains, It Pours

It wasn't until the second week of March that my cough from the norovirus finally cleared. Within a couple of days, I tested positive for COVID-19 again. When I updated my doctor, she issued another script for the earlier mentioned anti-viral medication. When I called the pharmacy to check if the prescription was ready, they informed me that the out-of-pocket price was over $1,000. After I picked up my phone from the floor, I told the pharmacy technician that I would not be picking up the script. As the infection ran its course, my COVID-19 infection cleared on its own with no adverse side-effects by the middle of March.

The March Races

I was signed up for two races in Chicago on March 23 and 24. The races were The Mile and the Shamrock Shuffle (8K). I had about a week to get some training in before driving to Chicago. I felt fully recovered from the norovirus and COVID-19; however, I knew that my fitness took a hit with all the time away from training.

The first race was The Mile. Upon arrival at the starting area, the race administrators announced a special guest in attendance, Galen Rupp. Mr. Rupp is an elite runner who represented the United States in the 2012 Olympic Games in London, winning the Silver Medal in the 10,000 meters with a time of 28:30, which averages to 4:25 MPM. The last time the U.S. won a metal in the Olympic 10,000 meters was in 1964, 48 years earlier. Five years later Mr. Rupp won the 2017 Chicago Marathon with a time of 2:09:20 (4:56 MPM), making him the first American to win since 2002 (worldmarathonmajors.com, 2025).

My goal was to beat my best time running the mile, which was 8:14. Running only one mile in a race was a new experience for me. On every other race I used the first mile as part of my warm-up. My best training time for a single mile was 9:08; so my goal was to break 8 minutes.

The race included a total of 422 runners, grouped into two waves—the elite wave and the recreational wave. I registered for the recreational wave, but when I saw a father and his son (under 10) lining up in the elite wave I decided to join them.

Once the race started, I established a sub-8 minute pace and my heart rate quickly rose to the mid-160s. The route oddly took us through a couple of 180° turns, which caused a slow-down. During the first half of the race I could feel the pace was taking a toll on me. I took a couple of very short walk breaks around the halfway mark. As I headed into the finish, I turned on the jets and noticed that Mr. Rupp was waiting at the finish line for each runner. I threw my fate to the wind and sprinted for the line. As I finished I received a congratulatory high-five and "Great job!" from Mr. Rupp. I was very pleased with a finish time of 8:11, and a new PR. Incidentally the boy and his dad finished ahead of me.

The Shamrock Shuffle (8K)

The following day was the Shamrock Shuffle 8K, which is the race that unofficially inaugurates the running season in Chicago. The turnout for this race was the polar opposite to The Mile, with many thousands of runners and walkers lined up to participate (Real Time Race Tracking, 2024).

My PR (and time to beat) going into this race was 53:42 (from 2022). In 2023 I ran this same race with my daughter, which was the first race of her life. We were not running that race for a particular time, but to finish together. This time I was running to set a new PR.

The day was cloudy with temperatures in the mid-thirties. I arrived wearing three-layers and ready for the brisk downtown Chicago winds. As is the case with these huge races, it took me time to reach the starting line. The race administrators released each of the corrals with a gap so as to reduce some of the inevitable crowding of runners that commonly occurs at the start of large races. My 5K split time was 32:31, which represents a pace of 10:28 MPM. I ran the final third at a 10:08 MPM and finished the race with a time of 51:23, a new PR by 1:19 (Real Time Race Tracking, 2024).

Returning from Chicago with two new PR times was gratifying, especially since I lost so much training time to illness. Running in colder temperatures turned out to be more pleasant than I realized. The cool wind helped regulate my body temperature, which naturally rises while I run.

Prostate Surgery in April

Earlier in the book, I referred to my enlarged prostate gland. The condition is called **benign prostatic hyperplasia**, or BPH for short. The prostate gland wraps around the urethra, which is the passage way that urine takes to leave the body. When the prostate is enlarged, it restricts the urethra, making urination difficult. The symptoms of BPH are progressively arduous and include difficulty with urination, waking up in the middle of the night to urinate, a weak stream during urination, and an increasing inability to completely empty the bladder (Mayo Clinic Staff, 2024). Any man with BPH knows exactly what I am talking about.

My BPH started developing in my late 40s, with mild symptoms. As the years passed, my symptoms steadily grew worse. In 2020 I scheduled an appointment with a local urology team. They suggested an implant procedure designed to pull the enlarged prostate tissue apart, thereby reducing the congestion on the urethra. I thought about the procedure and decided against it at that time.

Fast forward to January 2024. By this time, my BPH symptoms had worsened; so I made an appointment with a different urology team. This doctor presented an alternative treatment, called, the **Holmium Laser Enucleation of the Prostate**, or HoLEP. He explained that the HoLEP procedure was a permanent solution for BPH that removes some of the inner tissue of the prostate, which reduces pressure on the urethra. The recovery time after HoLEP is less than a week, which is significantly shorter than other BPH treatment options.

In February I was confirmed as a good candidate for HoLEP and on April 4 I underwent the procedure. By Monday, April 8 I returned to work. I was instructed to put running on hold for four weeks, however, my recovery went so well, I was permitted to resume running after just three weeks.

Living with the symptoms of BPH was difficult for me, but after undergoing the HoLEP procedure my quality of life greatly improved. Since the HoLEP surgery my urinary function has returned to normal, with no recurrence of BPH symptoms whatsoever.

15. Training in the Summer

My next race was scheduled for June 9, 2024 and was a half marathon in Chicago, called the Chicago 13.1®. The reason I enrolled in this race has a bit of a back story rooted in my interest in the Chicago Marathon.

In early 2024 I registered for the 2024 Chicago Marathon. The race administration sent me an e-mail rejection because my run time in the Columbus Marathon was not fast enough to qualify. Another way to obtain a race bib was to run the marathon on behalf of a charity. There were dozens of charities to choose from; so I made a list and contacted each of them for an opening. Most of the openings were already filled; however, a few had open spots. There was a catch. I needed to generate at least $1,200 in donations to the charity, with full payment being received by the charity before I would be provided with a marathon racing bib. I decided to look for another option.

On the Chicago Marathon website I read that if someone registers for all the sponsored races (The Mile, Shamrock Shuffle, and Chicago 13.1) then they qualify for the marathon. This is referred to as running the full Chicago race circuit. I didn't waste a second and registered for all the races except the marathon. I later discovered that the full circuit includes the Chicago marathon. In order to qualify as a full circuit runner, I needed to run the marathon from the previous season. Well, isn't that a catch-22?! After this discovery, I decided to abandon my 2024 Chicago Marathon aspirations.

Being born and raised in the Chicago area, I did not need anyone to twist my arm to run there, bringing to mind the old adage, "You can take the boy out of Chicago, but you can't take Chicago out of the boy."

The last half marathon race I had completed was in June 2023, called the Hometown Half, with the race location just a few miles from my home in Ohio. I completed this second half marathon with a time of 2:34:06, almost 16 minutes faster than the Columbus Half Marathon in 2022.

With the Chicago 13.1 being almost exactly one year after the Hometown Half, I planned to start training right after returning from my Chicago races in March. Due to my prostate surgery requiring three weeks of recovery, the remaining training time before the Chicago 13.1 would need to be focused and intentional.

Starting on April 25 I gradually resumed running, listening carefully to my body when it called for rest. The last thing I needed was any type of injury caused by an attempt to speed up the healing process or make up for lost time. Whatever fitness level I could gradually build over the next 5 weeks would be what I brought with me to Chicago.

Early Spring Heat

With the beginning of May came higher than normal temperatures, with daytime highs in the mid-80s Fahrenheit. Thankfully, my weekday training runs were early in the morning, often before sunrise. Saturday's long runs were hot.

I learned the benefit of a hat gator and arm sleeves. These clothing items provided a terrific sun shield for my arms, head, and neck. When the bright sun pounded down without these items, the heat seemed to burn the energy right out of me, regardless of how much water or other nutrition I was taking in.

I read several online posts on social media that spoke to the importance of some training in summer heat. This is sometimes referred to as heat acclimation, and just like any other aspect of training, it should be practiced. Training my body to face heat and higher temperatures gave me a first-hand experience of what I might be required to face during a race. Allowing my body to be familiarized with the effects of summer heat turned out to be very useful race preparation.

Remembering Kelvin Kiptum

As I mentioned earlier, the 2023 Chicago Marathon was the race that Kelvin Kiptum set a new world record. On February 11, 2024, just a few months after setting the record, Kelvin Kiptum and his coach died in a car accident in Kenya. Kiptum was only 24 years old, leaving behind a wife and two children (Karoney, 2024). The shock of his passing reverberated through the running world.

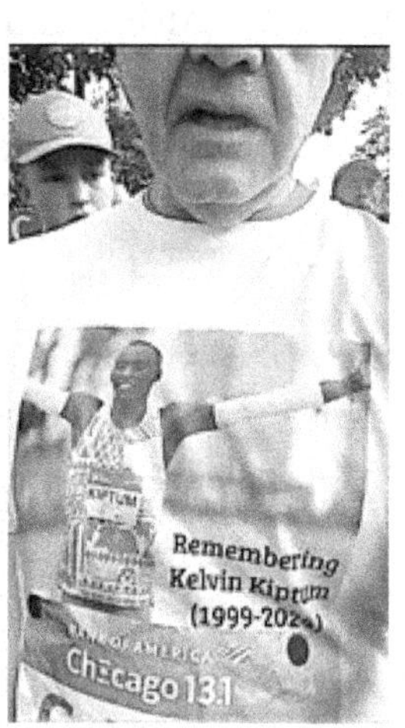

Photo by Bobby Schuler

I felt the need to honor this man in some way; so I had a T-shirt made with Kiptum's photo which I would wear during the Chicago 13.1 race.

The Chicago 13.1

When I drive from Columbus, Ohio to Chicago, Illinois it takes about six hours, not including the hour saved from the time zone change (from Eastern to Central). I thought to check pricing on a round-trip flight and to my surprise I found one that turned out to be slightly more than my round-trip cost for gas. The flight would bring me to Chicago O'Hare Airport two days before the race (June 7), with the return flight on the following Monday.

On the morning of the trip, the plane departed Columbus's John Glenn International Airport at 8:41 A.M. Eastern time and arrived in Chicago at 9:10 A.M. Central time. A massive improvement over six hours in the car. As the plane flew over Chicago, I

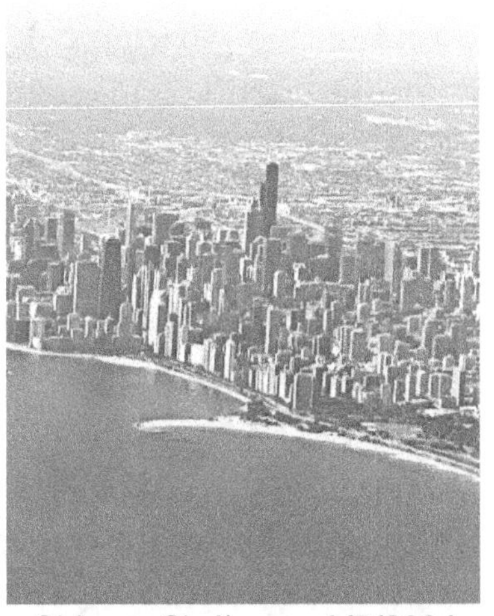

Chicago Skyline on 6/7/2024

snapped a photo from my window seat. I've always felt that Chicago's skyline ranks among the most beautiful in the world.

Once in the airport I boarded the Blue Line rapid transit train that conveniently took me downtown to obtain my race packet. I then walked over to the Metra (commuter) train station for a short ride to my daughter's apartment, located about 11 miles west of the city. I planned to stay with her for the duration of the trip. With it being the lunch hour and having about an hour before my train departure, I satisfied a craving for a Chicago hotdog from one of the shops located in the station's food court. It was not the best food for pre-race carbohydrate-loading, but it was delicious!

After arriving at the train station near my daughter's apartment I remembered that a running shoe store was located near the station. I walked in and asked a young man behind the counter if they carried a particular shoe that I had been eyeing for a while. The young man told me they did not have that shoe, but he did have a similar brand on sale. I asked to try them on and the shoes were remarkably comfortable. I liked the shoes so much that I walked out in them. I planned to use them for training when I returned to Columbus. I wasn't about to repeat the mistake I of running a race in new shoes, no matter how comfortable they felt. With a day and a half before the race, I looked forward to relaxation and rest.

Race Day—Chicago 13.1

On Sunday morning I followed my regular pre-race routine. My tapered training over the previous two weeks seemed to provide the perfect amount of race day preparation for my body to be in peak racing form. My goal was to beat 2:20, which would be a new PR.

My daughter drove me to the race with plenty of time to get situated in Corral C. The race location was on the near-west side of the city. As the crowds of participants steadily gathered, the total number was expected to exceed 10,000 runners. My thoughts about excessive heat were all for naught, as the morning temperatures were just under 60 degrees Fahrenheit, with low humidity and beautiful clear blue skies. As I moved toward the entrance of my corral, I passed long lines of people standing in front of many portable rest rooms. Thanks to my recent prostate surgery, I was grateful that I didn't need to join them.

As the race began I followed my plan to run 8 minutes and walk 1 minute. At the halfway mark my time was 1:10, which was aligned with the 2:20 target. As I began feeling the heat of the morning, I shortened the run portion to 4 minutes. I found a second wind near the end of mile 10, which continued into mile 11 and 12. It might have been due in part to the fun sign a spectator was holding that read, "On a scale from 1 to 10, you're a 13.1!"

With a mile left, I progressively pushed the pace through to the finish. My finishing race time was 2:21:59, just two minutes slower than my goal time, and a new PR.

After arriving home in Columbus I updated my run log and discovered that my run/walk ratio for the Chicago 13.1 was 84 percent (running) to 16 (walking). This showed a 14 percent increase in running over the Hometown Half Marathon that I ran a year earlier. Seeing this improvement in my fitness was very encouraging and affirmed to me that my body was responding positively to my training.

Another measurement of my running fitness is my VO2-Max number. A runner's VO2-Max is the measurement of the maximum amount of oxygen that a person can take into the body per minute when performing high-exertion exercise. In order to obtain a scientifically accurate VO2-Max test, it is best to be fitted with a mask in a controlled lab setting to measure exactly how much oxygen is consumed during the test (Sinurat, 2021). Many GPS running watches provide an estimated VO2-Max value that is calculated over time as run data is accumulated on the watch. This estimate has been found to be accurate to ±4%.

The VO2-Max number that my watch calculates is 43, which is between excellent and superior for a man in the sixties age group. This is another confirmation that my fitness is improving.

With the Chicago 13.1 now behind me, I created a three-week recovery plan to cover the remaining days of June. During this time I ran only 5Ks at an easy pace, with the exception of one progressively faster tempo run. During these recovery runs I kept a strict-focus to maintain HR zone-2. If my HR rose above 130 beats, I switched to walking until my HR was below 110 and then resumed my zone-2 run pace.

The Second 50K Plan

On July 1, 2024 I began an 18-week, 50K training plan, which ended on November 2, the day of the Chicago Lakefront 50K. This plan would not include a marathon training run, but I knew I would need a 20-miler. When thinking about finding a maximum training effort for my longest long run for the plan, I chose to place more emphasis on having enough fitness to complete the 50K. I settled in my mind that 20 miles would be my longest training run.

As the weeks passed and I progressed through my long runs, a 20-mile training run was scheduled for October 5. I attempted to complete the run, but became over-heated from high temperatures and cut the run short during mile 17. The following week I completed a 20-miler (on October 12), thanks to slightly cooler temperatures and starting the run well before sunrise. On a side note, my 1-mile loop route for the 20-mile training run took me past my neighbor's house over and over. Near the end of that run, maybe in mile 18, he jokingly called out to me from his yard, saying, "You can stop now, nobody is chasing you!" I responded, "I know! I'm chasing down type-2 diabetes!"

16. The Second Attempt

The last days of October 2024 were filled with anticipation of my second attempt at the Chicago Lakefront 50K race. I decided to drive to Chicago and my wife agreed to join me. We started the drive on Thursday morning, October 31, two days before the race, so that I would have a full day to load up on carbs and be ready to go early Saturday morning. I double-checked my gear pack before our departure and confirmed I had everything I needed before and during the race. This included sun protection, my hydration vest, my waist-band water bottles, and all the in-race nutrition that I tested during the summer training runs.

Race Morning

I rose during the four o'clock hour on Saturday, November 2, 2024. The morning was cool, but not as cool as the year before, with clear skies and pre-sunrise temperatures in the upper-forties Fahrenheit. Before leaving the hotel room, I stepped on the bathroom scale which reported a compact 156 pounds. My pant size was now 30-30 and my A1C was 5.9 (slightly above the normal range). After taking in some carbs at the hotel continental breakfast, we departed for the race location.

Upon arrival at the Foster Avenue boathouse

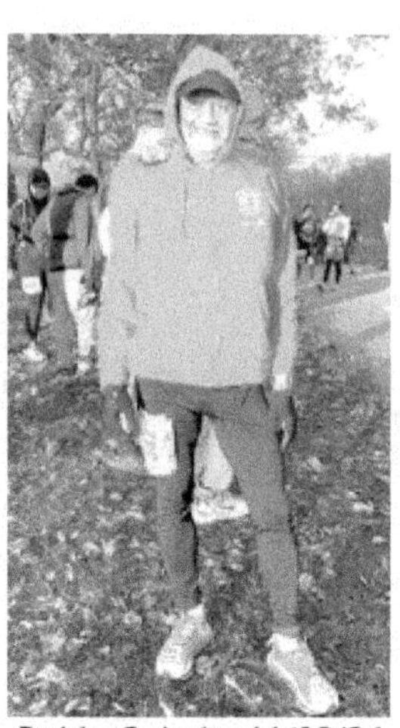

Bobby Schuler 11/02/24

we discovered that the 50-mile racers were already on the course. After checking in at the registration tent, I received my bib number and ankle timing module. The year earlier, my bib number was 420; this year I wore 342. The turnout was similar to last year with about 100 people registered for the 50K.

My taper phase started on October 13, the day after the 20-mile training run. My body felt very prepared. After doing some stretches and a short shake-out run I was ready to go. A few minutes before the start, I took my wife's hands in mine and she verbalized a prayer that no matter the outcome I would do my best and no one in the race would be injured.

This time, instead of lining up in the front I assumed my usual spot at the rear of the pack.

As the race began, I started the run app on my watch and kept my pace in check.

The day was stunningly beautiful with several sail boats still moored in Belmont Harbor. I arrived at the North Avenue turnaround just under 60 minutes, clocking an average pace of 10:49 MPM. I was feeling very good and hydrated; so I ran through the checkpoint.

My run on the second leg of this first 10-mile lap felt equally good. As the morning sun rose, I began to feel its warmth. After running through the timing mall at the end of leg 2, the air temperature rose to the mid-50s Fahrenheit. Feeling hot, I decided to remove my hoody before initiating leg 3. My average pace for leg 2 was 11:36 MPM, almost a minute per mile slower than the first leg. I made a pit stop at our supply bag and took one of the pre-made PB&J sandwiches, washing it down with some electrolyte water, and promptly initiated leg 3.

I walked more during this leg, with my average pace slowing to 14:08 MPM. I was eager to stop at the North Avenue aid station, where I was warmly greeted by a cheerful, buff young man.

"What can I do ya for?" he declared.

I saw a large container of peanut-butter pretzel nibs and took a handful and then looked over at a large glass jar that appeared to have lemonade in it.

"Is that lemonade?" I asked.

The man said, "Nope! Pickle juice. Want some?"

I asked, "Any guarantee that I won't puke it on the sand?"

He replied, "If ya do, enjoy it!" He went on to tell me that he completed his last 100-mile race drinking a lot of pickle juice. *His last 100-mile race?* I thought. That implied that he had run at least one other 100-mile race.

I accepted a small cup (maybe 4 ounces) and slugged it down. It tasted salty and better than I expected. I thanked him and resumed the race. Within a short time, I began to feel rejuvenated. It was like wonder juice.

My run/walk cadence on leg 4 was about 50/50 now and the lightness of the hydration vest indicated that I would need to add water when I completed this leg. Upon arrival at the Foster Avenue turn around, my body felt tired, but thankfully there was no pain in my knees or feet, like last time. After adding the water in my vest, I accepted another PB&J from my wife and softly told her, "One more lap, Sweety."

A Dark Place of the Mind

I felt significant fatigue as I started leg 5 and decided to walk mile 21. My brain compared my fatigue to the number of remaining miles in the race. I recalled my decision to cap my longest training run to 20 miles and wondered if it helped or harmed my fitness at this moment. Realizing that this line of thinking was useless, I refocused my thoughts on maintaining a good walking pace and occasionally testing my ability to resume running.

It must have been about a half mile into this leg that my brain completed its earlier calculations and began a process of negotiations. My thoughts seemed to say, *Your wife is less than a mile back there. All you have to do is turn around and tell her that you did your best, but completing a 50K race was just not in you today. She'll understand. Just stop now and call it quits.*

I recall seriously considering my mind's proposal and then offered an alternate perspective: there might not be too many opportunities for me to complete a 50K race after today. I was already two-thirds done and chose to keep walking forward. The farther I walked, the less persuasive the quit proposal became.

The Last Aid Station

I pulled into my last time at the North Avenue turnaround and headed straight to the table with the pickle juice. There were only a few people at the table now; so I asked if the man I saw earlier was still there so I could tell him how great the pickle juice was.

"Do you know his name?" one man asked.

I replied, "No, I don't know his name, but he told me he completed a 100-mile race."
A different man replied, "We all have completed multiple 100-mile races." The feeling of being out of my league returned.

I told them how much the pickle juice helped me. They stared back at me with a slow, affirming nod while I asked for a cup and then another. I drank at least 10 ounces of pickle juice this time, lingering at the fueling station to take in as much high-carb treats as I could.

One of the 100-mile guys standing nearby asked me, "Shouldn't you get going?" I downed a couple more pretzel nibs, thanked them all for their support and was on my way.

I began leg 6 with a walk, giving my digestive system time to process the fuel I had just taken in. Within a hundred meters I was in a gentle jog and feeling the pickle juice doing its marvelous work. Less than half a mile farther my watch vibrated with a message that read, "Congrats!! You just completed a new personal record in the Marathon! 6:01:45." I felt a wave of gratitude wash over me. Now, with every step, I was conquering a new distance, en route to completing, yet again, the longest race of my life.

A Friendly Gentleman

About another mile up the path I happened upon a gentleman around my age, walking in the opposite direction. He saw my race bib and asked me which race I was running. I told him and he smiled while shaking his head no and mentioned that it was incredible. He asked how far I had left. I told him that I just passed the marathon point. His no head gesture changed to a slow nod. He said, "Wow! I could never run a marathon, let alone an ultramarathon. You're doing great!"

It's amazing how powerful a simple word of encouragement can be when spoken at just the right time and in just the right context. This man's words renewed confidence in me, like taking in verbal pickle juice. While I still had miles to complete, this gentleman's words lifted my spirits. There are times, I believe, that God brings people across our path to encourage us exactly when we need them most.

A Sudden Threat

While the pickle juice from the aid station helped a lot, the fatigue in both my legs was significant. I was in a gentle jog and without any warning a muscle on the inner part of my left leg began to seize. I characterized the level of discomfort to the rumblings of an 8.5 Richter scale earthquake. It was as if my leg was saying, "If you continue jogging, I will unleash a charley horse upon you, the likes of which you have never felt before!" In an immediate attempt to deescalate the situation, I slowed to a walk and stretched the leg in different directions to see if I could loosen the tightness. Now walking, the muscle discomfort rapidly subsided, like that of a perfect decrescendo of a world-class orchestra under the direction of a virtuoso conductor.

With the muscle appeased, I continued walking, slowly increasing my pace while being mindful not to unnecessarily provoke my leg's earlier threat. Without experiencing any further pain I established a reasonably quick walking pace, while giving the suspect muscle as much time as it needed to recover, similar to a football player who just had the wind knocked out of him.

The Silent Biker

It was the 2 o'clock hour now, and more folks were on the trail enjoying the beautiful afternoon. With all my focus on my walk cadence and paying close attention for any objections from my leg, I didn't notice that I drifted to the left edge of the running lane. All of a sudden without a sound a cyclist in the tuck position on tri-bars, riding what looked like the most expensive bike I ever saw, *Z-I-P-P-E-D* past my left shoulder doing at least 25 mph. The instant blast of displaced air between us abruptly pushed me toward the center of my lane. After regaining my composure from the shock, I thought, *After all this, I almost get run over by a biker?* I instantly adjusted my walk line to the furthest from the bike lane.

Anomalous Thoughts Continue

I glanced down at my watch to see that I was in mile 28. With my walk cadence strong and my line away from the bikes, I found my-self only inches away from the blueish-green waters of Belmont Harbor. The water was gen-tly rising and falling, as if taking breaths in and out. A thought drifted in my mind: *Look at how cool the water looks. All you have to do is jump in. You'll be fine. Go ahead.* It was as if some hidden enemy was sitting on my shoulder taunting me. This suggestion was not as tempting as the quit proposal during mile 21. It reminded me of the Bible passage in chapter 4 of the book of Matthew, where Satan tempted Jesus to throw himself down from the pinnacle of the temple. I promptly quickened my walking pace, inten-tionally directing my steps toward the upcoming turn in the path and away from the water's edge.

A Familiar Voice

I was now in the final mile of the race and was taking the last turn onto the familiar gravel area where the race started over 7 hours earlier. With the finish in sight, I quickened my walking pace even more. I was not feeling any objections from my body, but was not ready to break into a run yet. To my pleasure, I heard a familiar voice in the distance: "I've got a visual!!" It was my son, who had joined my wife at the finish line. I continued walking and my son ran over to join me. He asked, "How are you feeling, Dad?" I told him I felt great and I wanted to jog into the finish. I caught sight of my wife, who was standing a few hundred feet ahead and applauding. The muscle in my left leg yielded to the elation of the moment, and did not bring up the earlier charley horse threat. My son joined me in the final jog and we crossed the finish line together.

Shortly after crossing, my watch vibrated with another notification, this one reading, "Chicago Lakefront Ultra—Fall (50K)." My official time was 7:33:29, placing me ninety-third out of 114 participants. With this being the first ultra race I completed, the race administrators gave me a commemorative glass with the embossed words, *I Survived My First Ultra.*

In the days following the race I discovered that all the race finishing times were published in Ultra Running Magazine®. I felt astounded, grateful, and amazed all at the same time.

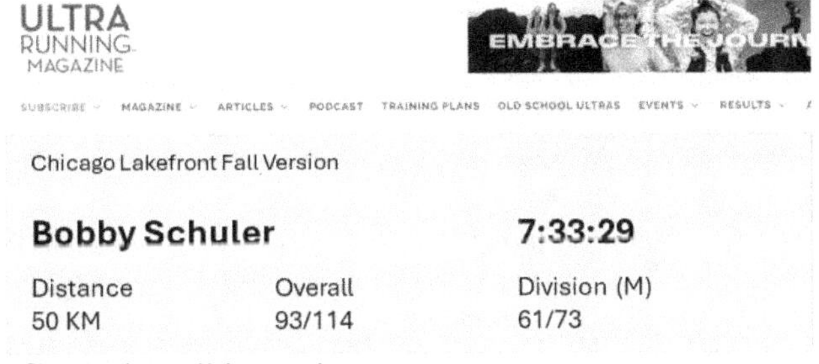

Chicago Lakefront Fall Version

Bobby Schuler   7:33:29

Distance	Overall	Division (M)
50 KM	93/114	61/73

Source: https://ultrarunning.com

17. What's happening in the Brain

In this chapter we will spend a few moments reviewing brain function. It may seem like too much info, but bear with me, as we will cover fascinating operations and interactions of the brain and how they help us with difficult tasks.

As I looked back over the endurance-building phases leading into my longest training runs and races, a question formed in my mind: What is really happening when my mind tells me it's time to quit? I'm not talking about being injured, like my knees and heel during my first 50K attempt. I mean during mile 21 of the second 50K attempt when my body was fatigued but uninjured. My mind was almost demanding that I stop and return to my wife. Why were those thoughts so persuasive to the degree that I almost quit the race?

In my search for answers I discovered a set of fascinating interactions involving a particular region of the brain that is activated almost exclusively when we attempt difficult and prolonged tasks. So let's get into it.

The Limbic System of the Brain

The **limbic system** (LS) is the part of the brain that assesses emotionally-charged situations we encounter. The LS regulates emotions, memory, and survival responses in difficult situations. An important part of the LS, is the **amygdala**, which is involved in processing emotions, especially fear. If we encounter a frightening experience, it is the amygdala that prompts a fight, flight, freeze, or fawn response to that experience (Yeschek, 2025). *Figure 6* displays different regions of the brain (Becker, 2019).

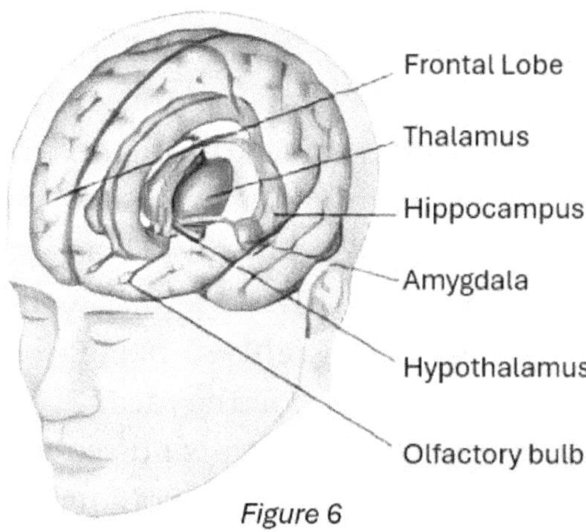

Figure 6

In the case of experiencing prolonged fatigue, such as competing in a marathon, the amygdala provides reasoning with the intention of guiding us away from suffering and back to **homeostasis**, that is, the calm state of equilibrium between body and mind that is safe from threats (Merriam-Webster's Medical Dictionary, 2016). The **hypothalamus** is a gland near the amygdala that passes messages from the body to the pituitary gland, which in turn releases various hormones, many of which help bring the body into homeostasis (Sutton, 2022, p. 197). The **hippocampus** is involved in the formation, processing, and storage of memories, bonding any emotional intensity associated with those memories (Merriam-Webster's Medical Dictionary, 2016).

The **anterior mid-cingulate cortex** (aMCC) is located near the frontal lobe and is an intersection point for several networks in the brain. The aMCC integrates signals from other brain systems to anticipate energy needs for attention and physical movement all toward the objective of achieving goals. (Touroutoglou et al., 2020). In contrast to the amygdala's goal to achieve homeostasis, the aMCC seeks to bring **allostasis**, or the state of internal and physical equilibrium when facing stressors (Merriam-Webster, 2025). The brain can be trained, through the activation of the aMCC, to find improved cognitive control, sensory perceptions, and motor functions when facing difficult physiological tasks (Touroutoglou et al., 2019).

Input from Experienced Brain Practitioners

My introduction to brain function came from friend and counselor Steve Yeschek. Steve is a licensed grief and trauma counselor with over 20 years of experience helping patients recover from trauma, including those suffering from varying degrees of post-traumatic stress disorder (PTSD).

Steve told me that the **prefrontal cortex** (PFC), located in the frontal lobe, is central to higher-order thinking such as decision-making and the regulation of emotions. Those who choose to calmly assess a perceived threat are engaging their PFC, which provides a platform for them to think clearly and face their situation rationally (Yeschek, 2025). Alternatively, an individual can choose to make decisions based on emotional inputs. When a threat is encountered, the amygdala offers a purely emotional response to the threat, with the only goal to find safety. This can lead to unclear thinking, often fueled by fear, and opens the door to negative thoughts. Steve shared that when a patient relives the experience of a trauma, his or her amygdala is over ruling his or her PFC. Additionally, the amygdala does not have cognitive ability; so it cannot distinguish between a past experience or a present threat. (Yeschek, 2025).

Steve introduced me to another brain practitioner, neuro-biofeedback specialist, Ed Epstein. Mr. Epstein is a brain fitness coach and a 10-41 advocate neuro-bio specialist with over 27 years of experience analyzing patient brain function. Ed studied and worked under the late Dr. Phillip S. Epstein, a graduate of the University of Chicago's division of biological sciences and the Pritzker School of Medicine, specializing in psychiatry, diagnostic radiology, and neurology (Epstein, 2025).

Ed told me that the amygdala is located in the lower brain region and requires training. When a person encounters a perceived threat, the response from an undisciplined amygdala is like "walking into a flooded basement" or "driving into an active warzone." The body's senses are on alert and tend to be dominated by negative self-talk that includes *I can't, I won't*, and *I will not*. Ed illustrated further that when the amygdala dominates one's thinking, "it's as if your brain has been hijacked [by negative forces], which hinders a person's ability to think clearly and calmly" (Epstein, 2025). Ed expounded that those who engage their upper brain (their PFC) are able to face challenges from a calm, clear-thinking perspective. This is because the PFC is the seat of higher-order cognitive functioning, decision-making, and emotional regulation (Epstein, 2025).

Limbic System and PFC Interaction

Clinical psychologist and therapist, Dr. Corky Becker asserts in her article, "The Neurobiology of Threat," that the PFC enables us to "create a sense of self, develop insight, empathy, and form moral judgments." The PFC is the area that enables us to pause before we act, to reflect, and to focus our attention (Becker, 2019).

Becker adds that the LS "gives meaning to our feelings" through the ability to trigger fearful memories (interaction between the amygdala and the hippocampus). She states that when the LS senses a perceived threat, it sends alarms that influence how we feel, think, and act. If the perceived threat is confirmed as a viable danger, then the LS can override the PFC and shut it down (Becker, 2019).

When I think back to mile 21 of my second 50K attempt I can distinctly remember stopping, turning around, and taking a few steps back toward my wife, then stopping again. In that moment my limbic system was making an attempt to shut down my PFC and persuade me to quit the race.

The aMCC and Tenacity

In February 2020, Massachusetts General Hospital and the Harvard Medical School conducted a study that showed "the aMCC is an important network hub in the brain that performs computations necessary for tenacity." The study proposes that the aMCC "integrates signals from diverse brain systems to predict energy requirements for attention allocation . . . and physical movement." The study suggests, in cooperation with other studies, that the aMCC is involved in "educational achievement, exercise, successful aging, and [can assist in the treatment of] neuropsychiatric disorders such as depression and dementia" (Touroutoglou et al., 2020).

In an online article on the importance of the aMCC, certified ELDOA® practitioner and level-3 CHECK practitioner T. J. Pierce shares that when we engage in physical activities, especially those that we find challenging or unpleasant, the aMCC is activated. It then grows and "enhances our ability to tackle stressful situations, improves our capacity for self-discipline, and boosts our overall cognitive function." Pierce states that we develop our aMCC when we engage in activities that are beneficial to us but that we do not enjoy doing. When we avoid those same activities, our aMCC shrinks and we forfeit the benefits that it provides to us (Pierce, 2024).

A Plan for Facing Difficulty

As I trained and raced in longer distances, I stretched out my body's resources which naturally caused fatigue and energy depletion. I always understood that attempting a half marathon, full marathon, or 50K ultra marathon would be difficult. When I think back to when I participated in those race distances for the first time, I experienced degrees of physical difficulty, even suffering. I had no idea that running would also bring mental battles.

I recalled three situations that exemplified the combination of fatigue, depletion, and mental battles:

- Hitting the wall during the Columbus Marathon (chapter 10),
- Struggles completing the 20-mile training run (chapter 15),
- Mental quit proposal during the second 50K race (chapter 16).

As I thought through the commonalities of these events, I discovered predictable elements that repeated during most of my long runs:

(1) Heightened levels of fatigue.

(2) Depletion of energy reserves.

(3) Knowledge that I was not physically injured.

(4) A mental battle between my limbic system and my PFC (that is, my amygdala seeking homeostasis versus my aMCC that offers allostasis).

New Preparation Steps

These four elements prompted me to adopt a new set of preparation steps before long runs and races. I wanted to be more aware of the expectation of physical fatigue, energy depletion, and thoughts that conflict with my race goals. Before any long run or race I intentionally decided to keep the following concepts in the forefront of my thinking:

1. I will have confidence in completed training and recovery. I will remind myself that I completed all planned training and recovery for this run or race (provided I actually did complete the training). I will fully-engage my body, mind, and soul to be ready to perform the training run or race to a successful conclusion, in accordance with my goal(s) for the training run or race.

2. I will follow a recovery, hydration, and fueling plan. I will plan all in-race recovery, such as taking walk breaks and having water and other nutrition readily available for the training run or race.

3. I will be prepared for injury or emergency. If a physical injury occurs during the run or race, I will acknowledge it, assess the severity, and calmly decide if I am able to continue. If a circumstance arises that poses a threat apart from a running injury, I will set aside my race goal(s), listen to guidance from race administration, and choose a safe course of action.

4. I will manage thoughts and internal dialogue. I will evaluate every thought that enters my mind, positive or negative. If any thought contradicts my goal(s) for the training run or race, apart from any of the above three steps, or presents an irrational idea or fear, I will challenge that thought. I will not allow a race-ending decision to be made solely on emotional input.

The possibility always exists that I will encounter an event or situation outside my control. I had to learn that these situations are truly not worth worrying about or wondering why they happen—like the "sharp poke" I felt in my shoe during the Columbus Marathon. My new steps provide me with a reasonable plan to keep fatigue, depletion, injury, and anomalous thoughts in check. By continuing through difficulty (including some measurement of non-injury suffering), my new steps bring a reasonable expectation to receive cognitive and tenacious assistance from my brain (allostasis) to overcome the difficulty and achieve the goal(s) I set for my training and races.

These steps are useful not only in my training and race competitions, but for addressing all types of challenges in all areas of my life. Not all challenges cause physical fatigue and depletion, but other challenges may cause emotional and relationship fatigue. It is always useful to remind myself that it is not my place to attempt to control the thoughts, words, or actions of another person. I am responsible only for my own thoughts, words, and actions. I discovered that choosing to remain in a non-life-threatening situation and refraining from fight, flight, freeze, or fawn responses will cause my character (and brain) to grow, along with helping me avoid hurting others with impulsive, emotionally-charged words and actions. This path helps create new inner strength that aids in facing my own fears and apprehensions.

18. Bobby Schuler's Ten-Steps

It was after reviewing my training log following the completion of the 50K race that
I began to see a set of repeating patterns in
my training. After I realized that they totaled
ten steps, I decided to call them *Bobby Schuler's
Ten Steps for Training (Ten Steps)* see *Figure 7*.

The Ten Steps are enclosed in two repeating
loops; one loop that repeated steps 4, 5, and 6,

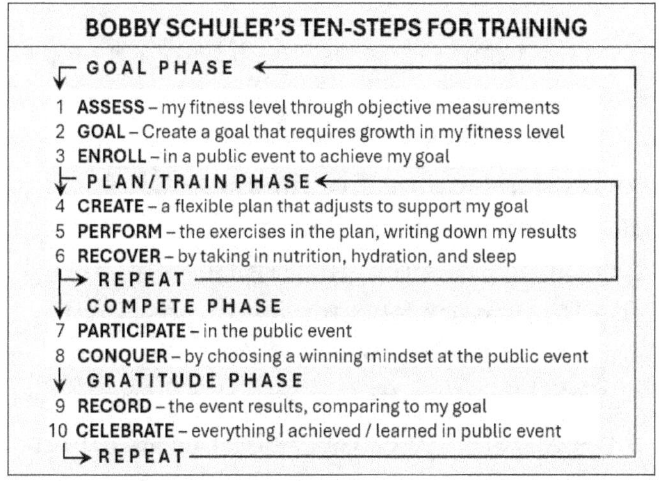

Figure 7

related to daily training, and the other loop repeating all Ten Steps for each new training

plan. The Ten Steps became my foundation for staying consistent in my training. I found that maintaining consistency was the most meaningful and substantive way that I achieved my goals and lasting results.

The Phases of the Ten-Steps

As shown in *Figure 7*, the Ten-Steps are organized into four high-order phases: (1) goal, (2) plan/train, (3) compete, and (4) gratitude. Let's take a closer look at each phase, and the steps within them.

The GOAL Phase

The goal phase is made up of steps 1 through 3.

Step 1, **Assess** (or assessment) is important for understanding my fitness level. A formal assessment is a test of specific movements, flexibilities, or strength performed by the exerciser to provide a healthcare professional with an idea of the physical ability of the exerciser. Gaining an objective assessment of my current physical ability can be obtained through a standardized test or from analyzing my recent training results (as recorded in my training log). My fitness level can also be influenced by time away from training caused by illness or other medical procedures that require that I pause my training. As soon as I have an understanding of my fitness level, I'm ready for the next step.

Step 2, **Goal** is the process of creating a fitness achievement that involves a challenge beyond my current fitness level. Often enough I could create a goal based on recently completed race finish times or distances. If I chose a speed goal I would cap the increase to 5% faster than my fastest previous time. If my goal involved running a new distance for the first time, then I often set my goal to finish the race without a time goal. Once the race was completed I could then use that race time as my baseline for the next time I ran that race distance.

Step 3, **Enroll** is signing up for a public event in the future that allows for enough training time to prepare my body to achieve the goal. On several occasions I completed steps 2 and 3 interchangeably because I found a race to my liking that stretched my ability and then set a goal for it.

The PLAN/TRAIN Phase

The plan/train phase includes steps 4 through 6.

Step 4, **Create** involves building a training plan around the public event that I registered for in step 3. In the early stages of my training when preparing to run my first half marathon, I didn't know how to build a training plan; so I took the advice of Hal Higdon and used one of his novice plans as a starting place. I'm always open to reviewing a training plan authored by a seasoned runner or a professional coach. Using a training plan is intended to be a guide to my training and is not set in concrete. I need to be open to listening to my body and taking into account my stress level, in addition to knowing the quality of my recovery and sleep. I focus on being flexible enough to allow an occasional adjustment to the plan.

Step 5, **Perform** is the actual execution of the exercises in the plan. This step repeats each day, as defined in the training plan. I prefer to train early in the morning. Once the training is completed, then the key statistics from that training session are updated in my training log. Keeping up-to-date records of my training sessions allows me to see my progress, along with being a source of encouragement.

Step 6, **Recover** involves food, hydration, and sleep. This step is just as important as Step 5, and when I follow it well, I see the maximum benefits from my training. It includes taking in adequate macro-nutrients (carbs, proteins, and lipids) along with sufficient water and electrolytes before, during, and after training. Receiving quality sleep is an important part of my recovery.

The COMPETE Phase

The Compete phase is my favorite phase in the Ten Steps. This is the phase that applies all the built up fitness to a public event.

Step 7, **Participate** is the step that starts with the day or two of rest just before the public event, following the completion of the taper phase on the training plan. Anticipation is building for me during this step because I know that the public event is the next time I will exercise. The night before the event involves a carb-loaded meal with plenty of water, loading my car with whatever is needed, and setting out my racing clothes for the event.

Step 8, **Conquer** is the step where my competitive side is on full display. Once that race horn sounds, my mind shifts all attention to the goal(s) during the race combined with a continual sensing of how my body is performing during the event. Most of the time I am competing against my last best time or am focused on completing a new furthest distance that I had yet to complete. Occasionally though, I will see someone ahead of me as I approach the finish, and I'll sprint to beat him in the last seconds of the race.

The GRATITUDE Phase

The Gratitude phase is the part where I record all the event results in my log. This phase is also about being thankful for all the support I received from my family and all involved in the event.

Step 9, **Record** involves reviewing and capturing all that I accomplished during the public event. This usually involves reviewing the running metric data captured on my watch, but can also include other types of accomplishments, such as a PR time or a first-ever race distance being completed.

Step 10, **Celebrate** is fairly self-evident. My celebrations often involve having a special meal after the event or posting a photo on social media. In the days following the event, my thoughts often drift to the question, *What's next?* This leads me to the word **Repeat** at the bottom of *Figure 7*, which has a long, arrowed line that wraps around all Ten Steps and back to the goal phase to start the process over with a new goal and a new event.

Since I started consistent training I feel more energetic and less random aches and pains. I also noticed that I think quicker. I've seen postings on social media from others who experienced the same. When I look at the key words for the first six steps, I noticed they form acronyms (*Figure 8*).

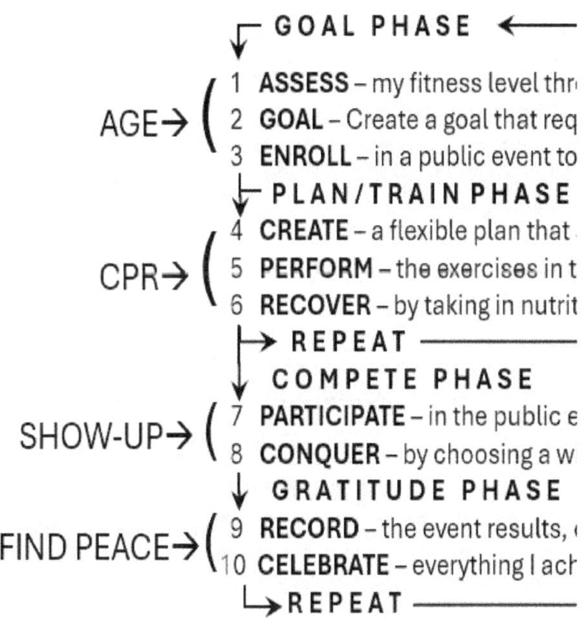

Redefining AGE

The goal phase is made up of the first three steps, assess, goal, and enroll. The first letter of these key words forms the word *AGE*. By following these steps for every training plan I started, I was in essence redefining what the word age meant to me. It was no longer only the number of years accumulated since my birth. To me the word AGE was now expanded to mean:

(1) A process for understanding my current health status.
(2) Boldly reaching for new goals and growing my abilities.
(3) Enrolling in public events and competitions with other health-conscious people.

A New Kind of CPR

Steps 4 through 6 contain the words create, perform, and recover, which form the acronym CPR. Since starting my first training plan back in 2022 for the Columbus Half Marathon, I learned that having a plan breathes life into my goals. Creating a plan is similar to my car. The power from the engine must be delivered to the wheels (via the transmission and differential). The benefits from training builds fitness that delivers energy to my body through the creation, performance, and recovery of a structured training plan. This new CPR means:

(1) Intentionally thinking about what my body needs and creating a plan that directly addresses those needs.

(2) Performing exercises in the plan with commitment and dedication.

(3) Treating proper nutrition, hydration, and sleep as equal elements to support my health and vitality.

As I follow these six initial steps I am defining my abilities by my performance, not by any limit associated with my chronological age. I maintain a level-head by setting goals within a reasonable and achievable range. When my goals are challenging me, I can expect that my aMCC (the anterior mid-cingulate cortex) will grow. I understand that this improves the functioning of my brain, which helps me stay focused on completing my goal(s)—and helps me be useful to the people in my sphere of influence.

The Final Four Steps

Step 7 and Step 8 are the **show-up** steps. When I thought back to my first race, the duathlon (see chapter 2), there was a moment when I thought to myself, *There is no turning back now. I'm doing this!* I expected to clock one of the slowest times. Showing up to an event requires courage and a willingness to put myself out there in front of others. For me that often involved humility. Humility is good, because it causes us to grow.

The gratitude phase in Step 9 and 10 allows me to **find peace** by finding thankfulness in all that I accomplished from the previous 8 steps. This includes cheering on others who pushed themselves to grow into a better version of themselves.

A Higher Quality of Life

By following my Ten Steps, I have discovered a higher quality of life through the daily use of my muscles, tendons, ligaments, and cardiorespiratory system. To me, choosing to train brings mobility and strength that enables me to do more and be more useful to others.

Concluding Thoughts

My original goal with exercise was focused on beating type-2 diabetes. I knew that an exercise program would be a big part of that effort. The program needed to be simple and geared for a beginner. The program also needed to help lower my elevated B/G levels. Through my Ten Steps, I discovered a blueprint that anyone desiring to improve their health could follow and begin enjoying the benefits of daily movement and a more active lifestyle.

I understand that this book speaks a lot about the sport of running. Running happens to be the mode of exercise that best meets my health needs. I want the core message of this book to be my encouragement to you to take heart and begin your own search for an exercise program that meets your health needs and can provide you with the joy that comes from daily movement.

Postlude

As I established a daily run training routine, it was not all cheers and accolades. When I shared my running goals and accomplishments with friends, most were encouraging but some responded with resistance. They were concerned that I was too old for strenuous exercise. Maybe there's a part in all of us that struggles with the idea that an older adult can participate in long races or lift heavy weights. From a statistical perspective it is easy to understand this opinion. How many men in their 60s set a goal to complete a first ever half marathon, full marathon, or ultramarathon? Not many.

I found this resistance very motivating. With every new distance or race that I completed I affirmed that I was capable. I used each successful workout and race to mentally fuel my next challenging goal. At the same time, I reminded myself that my choices and behaviors were responsible for me developing type-2 diabetes and I am <u>the only person</u> who could do anything about it. No one else could exercise for me. With each completed workout I believed that my efforts were gradually making me into a new person. Even at my age, I discovered that new beginnings are possible.

Today I see myself through a new lens with new capabilities. I see myself as a runner, weightlifter, competitor, and an endurance athlete. In the beginning I felt inadequate and overwhelmed. I slowly began to realize that part of my training involved changing my thinking from "How can I?" to "I will!"

My goal with this book is rooted in the hope that what I shared of my journey will inspire others to find their own reason to begin a progressive plan for daily movement. It was not easy for me to start, but as I continued taking simple steps in manageable daily chunks I was able to find enough courage each day to follow my plan. I discovered that taking those simple steps one day at a time was the best way to stay consistent. I did not know that those simple daily steps would lead me to extraordinary results.

A Plan Requires a Design

When I studied computer programming in college I learned how to process data through the execution of different coding techniques. My programs needed to be meticulously planned and designed with a specific purpose in mind in order to achieve the required output. This process never happened by chance. If I mistyped a key word in a program or loaded incorrect data in a controlling variable, the resulting output would be incorrect and sometimes disastrous.

My programs included varying degrees of complexity. I often pondered more complex processes, such as the manufacturing of an automobile, which involves the integration of thousands of machined, electronic, plastic, and sheet metal parts that are designed to function together in harmony. Most cars that are driven daily last less than fifteen years and then need to be replaced.

As I mentioned at the beginning of this book, human beings are living longer, many past 100 years. Doctors and scientists the world over are constantly making new discoveries about the human body, proving over and over that its complexities remain far beyond man's complete knowledge.

With all this said, it is my belief that the human body came about by the intelligent design of God. I acknowledge that physical exercise and daily movement are limited in the benefits they provide. Even the Bible states that ". . . bodily exercise has some value, but godliness has value in all things, having the promise of the life which is now and of that which is to come" 1 Timothy 4:8 (World English Bible, 2020). With these words, I hear a call to care for my body, being willing to use it to glorify God through service to others, while I live, and move, and have my being.

You Are Special

Below is a publication that speaks to the uniqueness and value of each human person. These words were written by Ted Griffin and wax eloquent on this topic, reprinted here with permission from the author (GRIFFIN, 2023):

> "There are no ordinary people. You have never talked to a mere mortal," wrote C. S. Lewis. It's true—each one of us is a special creation of God.
>
> Believe it or not—no one else is just like you. Your physical appearance, your voice and personality traits—your habits, intelligence, personal tastes—all these make you one of a kind. Even your fingerprints distinguish you from every other human being—past, present, or future. You are not the product of some cosmic assembly line; you are unique.

But the most important fact of your identity is that God created you in his own image (Genesis 1:27). He made you so you could share in his creation, could love and laugh and know him person to person. You are special indeed!

The Bible reveals God's total interest in you as an individual. The psalmist wrote in one of his most beautiful prayers, "I praise you, for I am fearfully and wonderfully made" (Psalm 139:14). God knew you even before you were born. Then, and now, he has plans just for you, plans conceived in love.

As we appreciate God's constant concern for us, we really begin to grasp the awfulness of sin. He loves you and me so much; yet how often we go our own way, turning our backs on him. God's designs for our lives are then blocked; his mercies do not come to the unwilling.

But even here we are precious to God, for he continues to love us even when we pay him no mind. He still sees us as individuals with great value. No wonder the psalmist declared, "How precious to me are your thoughts, O God!

How vast is the sum of them! If I would count them, they are more than the sand" (Psalm 139:17–18). God is not an unfeeling, cold-hearted monarch of the heavens. He feels our pains; he shares our sorrows. He cares, and he considers each one of us important enough to love.

In fact, he loves us so much that he gave his only Son to die for our sins. "In this is love," the Bible says, "not that we have loved God but that he loved us and sent his Son to be the propitiation [full payment] for our sins" (1 John 4:10).

Because you and I are special to God, he wants to forgive us and give us a full, meaningful life. When we trust in Jesus Christ and let him put our lives together, the Bible says that we become "God's masterpieces, created in Christ Jesus" (Ephesians 2:10, paraphrase). Can anyone be more special than that?

Yes, you are valuable to God! If you have never trusted Jesus Christ for your salvation, you can pray something like this today:

> Lord, thank you for sending Jesus Christ to die for my sins and rise from the dead so that I can know your forgiveness and live with you forever. Right now I ask him to be my Savior so that I can live as the special creation that you intended me to be."

I prayed a similar prayer during my college days and sensed a new beginning in my life. Since then, my life has not been perfect and I have made mistakes along the way. One thing was settled in my heart; that I knew that Jesus was with me, even in my worst moments and most challenging times.

An Anchor for the Soul

If you would like to know more about the Christian faith I encourage you to acquire the book *An Anchor for the Soul* by Dr. Ray Pritchard. This book explains what believing in Jesus is all about and answers common questions about the Christian faith. You can find this book on Amazon or via the website, keepbelieving.com.

Works Cited

American Pie Party, T. (2022, September 3). *https://runsig-nup.com/Race/OH/Hilliard/PediatricCancer5KPieRun*. https://runsignup.com/Race/OH/Hilliard/Pediatric-Cancer5KPieRun

Becker, C. P. (2019). *The neurobiology of threat.* https://whatisessential.org/sites/default/files/re-source/file/2019-11/Neurobiol-ogy%20of%20Threat.pdf

Burfoot, A. (2026). Jeff Galloway, Legendary Marathoner and Coach, Dies at 80. *Marathon Handbook.*

CDC. (2023). *Deaths by Select Demographic and Geographic Characteristics.* Https://Www.Cdc.Gov/Nchs/Nvss/Vsrr/Covid_week ly/Index.Htm#SexAndAge.

CDC. (2024, May 15). *Type 2 Diabetes.* Https://Www.Cdc.Gov/Diabetes/about/about-Type-2-Diabetes.Html. https://www.cdc.gov/diabe-tes/about/about-type-2-diabetes.html

Champion, Kate. (2020). *Never too late : inspiration, motiva-tion, and sage advice from 7 later-in-life athletes.* Mountain Morning Press.

Clark, Nancy. (2020). *Nancy Clark's sports nutrition guide-book.* Human Kinetics.

Cleveland Clinic, T. (2023). *Norovirus.* https://my.cleve-landclinic.org/health/diseases/17703-norovirus

Epstein, E. (2025). *Phone Interview with Ed Epstein.*

Fitzgerald, Matt. (2014). *80/20 running : run stronger and race faster by training slower.* Berkley.

Galloway, Jeff. (2016). *The run walk run method.* Meyer & Meyer Sport (UK) Ltd.

Goggins, D. (2024, May 25). *Your Mind Quits Way Before Your Body* [Video recording]. youtube.com. https://youtube.com/shorts/-pcQjdnH-Ho?si=Y3u0GmY9zwgywyQs

GRIFFIN, TED. (2023). *YOU'RE SPECIAL (ESV 25-PACK)*. CROSSWAY BOOKS.

He, S., & Sharpless, N. E. (2017). Senescence in Health and Disease. *Cell, 169*(6), 1000–1011. https://doi.org/10.1016/j.cell.2017.05.015

Higdon, H. (2025). *About Hal Higdon*. Https://Www.Halhigdon.Com/about-Hal-Higdon/. https://www.halhigdon.com/about-hal-higdon/

Higdon, Hal. (2016). *Hal Higdon's half marathon training*. Human Kinetics.

Higdon, Hal. (2020). *Marathon : the ultimate training guide : advice, plans, and programs for half and full marathons*. Rodale Books.

Karoney, C. (2024, February 12). *Kenyan marathon world record holder Kelvin Kiptum dies in road accident*. Https://Www.Bbc.Com/News/World-Africa-68270866. https://www.bbc.com/news/world-africa-68270866

Level Up Culture. (2022, November 24). *David Goggins: Hardest Man God Ever Created - A Level Up Culture Original* [Video recording]. youtube.com. https://www.youtube.com/watch?v=o28rtG31fdM

Mathis, David. (2025). *A little theology of exercise : enjoying Christ in body and soul*. Crossway.

Mayo Clinic Staff. (2024, September 24). *benign prostatic hyperplasia*. https://www.mayoclinic.org/diseases-conditions/benign-prostatic-hyperplasia/symptoms-causes/syc-20370087

Merriam-Webster. (2020). *Merriam-Webster's dictionary and thesaurus*. Merriam-Webster, Incorporated.

Merriam-Webster. (2025). *Mirriam-Webster Online Diction-ary*. Https://Www.Merriam-Webster.Com/. https://www.merriam-webster.com/

Merriam-Webster's Medical Dictionary, 865 (2016).

National Kidney Foundation. (2014). Diabetes and Your Eyes, Heart, Nerves, Feet, and KidneysNa. *Https://Www.Kidney.Org/Kidney-Topics/Diabetes-and-Your-Eyes-Heart-Nerves-Feet-and-Kidneys*. https://www.kidney.org/kidney-topics/diabetes-and-your-eyes-heart-nerves-feet-and-kidneys

New York Racing Association, Inc. , T., & Chic Anderson. (1973, June 9). *Secretariat - Belmont Stakes 1973* [Video recording]. youtube.com. https://youtu.be/AG_27cCW5bw?si=pMr1EqhvgCco1Wuf

Pierce, T. J. (2024, January 20). *The Challenge of Exercise*. Https://Piercefamilywellness.Com/Exercise-Brain-Function/. https://piercefamilywellness.com/exercise-brain-function/

Real Time Race Tracking. (2024a, March 23). *Bobby Schuler Finish Time - The MILE*. Https://Track.Rtrt.Me/e/BASS2024-MILE#/Tracker/R9H64ST7. https://track.rtrt.me/e/BASS2024-MILE#/tracker/R9H64ST7

Real Time Race Tracking. (2024b, March 24). *Bobby Schuler Shamrock Shuffle Finish*. Https://Track.Rtrt.Me/e/BASS2024#/Tracker/RRLZ94DN. https://track.rtrt.me/e/BASS2024#/tracker/RRLZ94DN

Romanov, N. S. ., & Robson, John. (2004). *Dr. Nicholas Romanov's Pose method of running : a new paradigm of running*. PoseTech.

Ruvolo, L. (2018). Louie Ruvolo X Profile. In *X. X.*

Schwarzenegger, A. (2023). *Arnold's Pump Club*. Schwarzenegger, Arnold. https://arnoldspump-club.com/

Schwarzenegger, A. (2026). *Arnold's Sports Festival*. Arnoldsports.Com.

Sinurat, R. (2021). Implementation Of The Evaluation Of The Volume Of Maximum Oxygen Uptake (Vo2 Max) Athletes Koni Rokan Hulu. *Jurnal Humanities Pengabdian Kepada Masyarakat*, 2(1). https://doi.org/10.24036/jha.0201.2021.01

Spielberg, Steven., Zanuck, R. D. ., Brown, David., Benchley, Peter., Gottlieb, Carl., Scheider, Roy., Dreyfuss, Richard., Shaw, Robert., Gary, Lorraine., Hamilton, Murray., Kramer, J. C. ., Backlinie, Susan., Butler, Bill., Fields, Verna., & Williams, John. (2012). *Jaws*. Universal Studios Home Entertainment.

Sutton, B. G. . (2022). *NASM essentials of personal fitness training*. Jones & Bartlett Learning.

Tinfang, R. M. , M. (2014). *Medical Phone Call*.

Touroutoglou, A., Andreano, J., Dickerson, B. C., & Barrett, L. F. (2020). The tenacious brain: How the anterior mid-cingulate contributes to achieving goals. In *Cortex* (Vol. 123, pp. 12–29). Masson SpA. https://doi.org/10.1016/j.cortex.2019.09.011

Touroutoglou, A., Andreano, J. M., Adebayo, M., Lyons, S., & Barrett, L. F. (2019). Motivation in the Service of Allostasis: The Role of Anterior Mid-Cingulate Cortex. In *https://doi.org/10.1016/bs.adms.2018.09.002 Get rights and content* (pp. 1–25). https://doi.org/10.1016/bs.adms.2018.09.002

Triregistration.com. (2021, September 26). *OFC Mini Du*. https://triregistration.com/TriResultsNew.php?raceid=4390

U.S. Census Bureau. (2018, March 18). *Older People Projected to Outnumber Children for First Time in U.S. History*. CB18-41.

https://www.census.gov/newsroom/press-re-
leases/2018/cb18-41-population-projections.html

USATF. (2025). *USATF - About Page.*
Https://Www.Usatf.Org/About.
https://www.usatf.org/about

Wolfe, R. R., Miller, S. L., & Miller, K. B. (2008). Optimal
protein intake in the elderly. *Clinical Nutrition, 27*(5),
675–684. https://doi.org/10.1016/j.clnu.2008.06.008

World English Bible. (2020). *World English Bible Online.*
Https://EBible.Org/Engwebu/1TI04.Htm.

World Masters Athletics. (2025). *What are the age categories
for Master Athletics?* https://world-masters-athlet-
ics.org/sp_faq/2197/

WorldAthletics.org. (2025). Https://Worldathletics.Org/.

worldmarathonmajors.com. (2025). *Galen Rupp, Jordan Ha-
say Among American Standouts for Bank of America Chicago Marathon.* Https://Www.Worldmarathonma-
jors.Com/Content-Hub/Galen-Rupp-Jordan-Hasay-
among-American-Standouts-for-Bank-of-America-
Chicago-Marathon. https://www.worldmarathonma-
jors.com/content-hub/galen-rupp-jordan-hasay-
among-american-standouts-for-bank-of-america-chi-
cago-marathon

Yeschek, S. (2025). *Phone Interview with Steve Yeschek.*

List of Figures

Recommended Reading

In addition to the books I referenced in this manuscript, the below works provided me with inspiration and guidance as I learned the training lifestyle:

Born to Run, by Christopher McDougall
Can't Hurt Me, by David Goggins
Do Hard Things, by Steve Magness
The Endurance Diet, by Matt Fitzgerald
Far Beyond Gold, by Sydney McLaughlin
Finding Ultra, by Rich Roll
Never Finished, by David Goggins
Older Faster Stronger, by Margaret Webb
Resilience, by Eric Greitens
Running The Dream, by Matt Fitzgerald

Acknowledgements

For the practical information I receive from their organizations:

Arnold's Pump Club (arnoldspumpclub.com)
Marathon Handbook (marathonhandbook.com)
National Academy of Sports Medicine (NASM)

For their valuable input on brain function:
  Ed Epstein and Steve Yeschek

For their input on all aspects of my health:

Paul Barnes	Matthew Lee, MD
Bob Boorman	Ray Pritchard, PhD
Susan Delman, MD	Matt Roby
Davis Duggins	Justin Ryan
Nancy Graesser, DO	Victor Santiago
Emily Ickes, APRN-CNP	Mike Sudermann
Al & Carol Kohn	R. M. Tinfang, MD

For their encouragement and belief in me:
  My wife and our adult children

To God, for pouring His love, mercy, and grace in my life through his Son and my Lord, Jesus Christ.

Index

About the Author

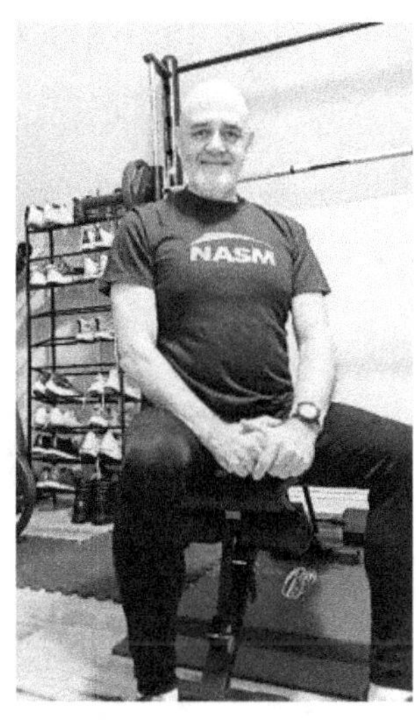 **Robert F. Schuler** is a certified personal trainer (CPT) and senior fitness specialist (SFS) through the National Academy of Sports Medicine (NASM). Prior to finding passion for fitness, Robert worked a 40-year career in technology and procurement. He is a graduate of Triton College, majoring in business and computer science. In addition to training and writing, Robert enjoys keeping up with his adult children, studying the Bible, learning new technologies, and enjoying music (especially the trumpet). He and his wife, Laura, reside in Ohio with their dogs, Milo and Nola.

You can follow Robert (listed as Bobby Schuler) on Strava or contact him via e-mail at:

BOBBYS10STEPS@GMAIL.COM